实用医疗英语

Practical Medical English

主　编　吴嫣斐　苏　娜
副主编　袁　芳　吴素芳　谢苑苑
编　委　徐宁骏　宓芬芳　朱莹莹　王　宇

U0249704

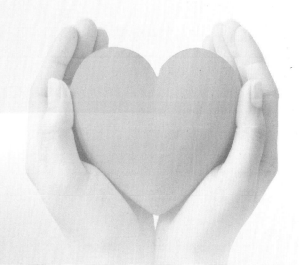

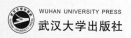

WUHAN UNIVERSITY PRESS

武汉大学出版社

图书在版编目(CIP)数据

实用医疗英语 / 吴嫣斐,苏娜主编 . -- 武汉 : 武汉大学出版社,
2024.12. -- ISBN 978-7-307-24644-7

Ⅰ.R

中国国家版本馆 CIP 数据核字第 20248QU974 号

责任编辑:吴月婵　　　责任校对:鄢春梅　　　版式设计:马　佳

出版发行:**武汉大学出版社**　　(430072　武昌　珞珈山)

（电子邮箱:cbs22@ whu.edu.cn 网址:www.wdp.com.cn)

印刷:武汉中科兴业印务有限公司

开本:787×1092　1/16　印张:20.25　字数:378 千字　插页:2

版次:2024 年 12 月第 1 版　2024 年 12 月第 1 次印刷

ISBN 978-7-307-24644-7　　定价:89.00 元

主编简介

　　吴嫣斐，女，浙江嘉善人，嘉兴大学外国语学院教师。瑞典布莱京理工学院英语语言文学硕士。长期从事医学英语教学与研究工作，具有丰富的教学经验和深厚的专业背景。致力于将现代信息技术与教育深度融合，推动医学英语教育的现代化和国际化。主持浙江省线上线下混合式一流课程：大学英语（医学）。曾参与多部教材编写，并在外研社"教学之星"大赛、浙江省高校教师教育技术成果比赛中多次获奖。

　　苏娜，女，广东普宁人，吉林大学外国语学院外国语言学及应用语言学专业硕士，博士在读。嘉兴大学平湖师范学院英语专业专任教师。在国内外杂志发表多篇核心论文，主持省部级教改课题一项，参与省部级和市厅级课题多项。主编《大学生英语听力》教材，出版专著一部。在教学竞赛中，曾获外研社"教学之星"大赛全国复赛一等奖、浙江省高校教师教育技术成果一等奖、浙江省微课教学竞赛二等奖。

前　言

　　在这个全球化不断加深的时代，医疗领域的国际合作与交流日益频繁。为了应对这一挑战和机遇，我们深感有必要推出一部实用性和专业性兼具的《实用医疗英语》教材，将语言学习和专业学习相结合，为学习者提供一个全面、系统的医疗英语学习平台。

一、编写理念

　　首先，编写本教材的初衷是帮助医学及相关专业的学习者提升与专业相关的英语语言能力，使学习者不仅能够掌握专业英语知识，而且能够在真实场景中有效运用英语进行沟通、学术交流以及处理国际医疗事务。为了实现这一目标，在编写本教材时我们注重理论与实践的结合，以英语的实际使用为导向，以培养学习者在医学专业领域的英语应用能力为重点。我们希望学习者通过学习本教材，能够在实际工作中灵活运用所学知识，提高工作效率和质量。我们深知传统的医疗英语纸质教材往往呈现形式比较单一，侧重于词汇和语法的学习，而忽略了实际场景的实践与应用。为了弥补这一不足，本教材采用新形态，将信息技术与教育深度融合，以适应互联网时代学习特性需求，满足国家、社会和学习者个人发展的需要。

二、教材特色

　　1. 突出立德树人，将课程思政融入专业教育。根据每个单元"量身定制"课程思政元素，潜移默化、润物无声地有机融入，使课程思政教育与专业知识教育协调同步、相得益彰。精准设计课程思政目标，使课程思政教学目标与语言教学目标有机衔接。将学科内容模块和课程思政内容模块有机融合，在传统的纸质内容和多模态的数字资源中合理融入德育元素，使学科内容和课程思政内容相辅相成。根据学习者当前的学习任务目标，充分考虑新形态教材纸质资料和多模态数字资源相结合的特点，提供不同类型、不同梯度的支架。

2. 任务驱动，注重实践应用能力培养。基于单元主题，每个单元设置提升医学英语语言能力的产出任务。同时，产出任务的设计也注重与实践应用相结合。通过模拟医患对话、设计医疗主题海报、撰写平行病历等多样化的教学活动，学习者不仅能够提高英语"听、说、读、写、译"的综合运用能力，还能在实际操作中掌握专业术语和表达方式。此外，教材还强调团队合作和跨文化交际能力的培养，鼓励学习者在完成任务的过程中学会与来自不同文化背景的医护人员和患者进行有效沟通。教材以其实用性和互动性，为学习者未来在国际医疗领域的职业发展奠定了坚实的语言基础。

3. 教学内容安排循序渐进，由浅入深，实现多元能力发展。教材从基础的医疗词汇和句型开始，逐步引入更为复杂的语言结构和专业概念，确保学习者能够在稳固的基础上迈向更高层次。通过分阶段的学习，学习者能够持续积累知识，同时提高运用英语进行专业沟通的能力。此外，教材内容涵盖广泛，包括日常医患交流、医疗文书写作、医疗健康宣传等多样化场景，旨在全面提升学习者的"听、说、读、写、译"各项语言技能。结合最新的教学理念和方法，本教材还注重培养学习者的批判性思维、跨文化交际和合作学习的能力，使其在医疗实践中更加游刃有余。

4. 以现代信息技术为支撑，赋能混合式教学。教学内容和信息技术深度融合，创造了一个富有互动性和沉浸感的学习环境。学习者可以通过线上网络资源进行自主学习，同时也能在线下与师生进行实时交流和讨论，有效弥补了传统教室教学的局限性。此外，教材还配备了丰富的多媒体材料，如与单元主题相关的视听材料、音频对话等，使得枯燥的专业术语和复杂概念变得生动易懂。教师利用这种混合式教学模式，不仅可以提高学习者的学习效率，激发学习动力，还为他们未来在医疗行业中运用信息技术打下了坚实的基础。

三、体系结构

《实用医疗英语》作为一部新形态大学英语教材，我们精心构建了八个单元，每个单元围绕一个特定的主题展开：疾病预防、健康生活、医疗体系、传统中医、心理治疗、医患沟通、叙事医学以及人工智能与医学。这些单元旨在全面覆盖医疗领域的关键环节和最新发展，为学习者提供一个系统的学习路径。

每个单元由四个部分组成，确保学习者能够从不同角度深入理解和应用医疗英语。第一部分"View the Medical World"采用视听材料，向学习者展示与单元主题相关的实际医疗场景。这不仅有助于学习者对主题有一个直观的认识，还能够激发他们的学习兴趣，为后续的阅读文章奠定坚实的基础。

第二部分"Read to Explore Medical Knowledge"包含两篇课文（Text A 和 Text B），这两篇文章虽然基于相同的主题，但各自从不同的视角进行探讨。这种设计使得学习者能够从多个维度丰富自己对单元主题的理解。课文内容涵盖了中外医疗实践的发展，有助于学习者了解不同文化背景下的医疗实践，拓宽视野，并促进其对各种医疗实践优缺点的深入思考，从而提升跨文化交际能力和思辨能力。

第三部分"Apply Medical English"分为 A 和 B 两个模块。A 模块提供了不同医疗场景下的医患对话实例，要求学习者与同伴一起模仿并创作类似的对话，以增强其实际应用能力。B 模块则根据单元主题，设计了口头或书面的实践应用产出任务，要求学习者独立或合作完成。这些任务旨在培养学习者的合作学习能力以及在医疗实践中的应用能力。

第四部分"Self-Assessment"与每个单元的学习目标相呼应，引导学习者在完成单元学习后进行自我评价。这一环节有助于学习者反思自己的学习过程，巩固所学知识，形成完整的学习闭环。

《实用医疗英语》通过其结构化和多元化的单元设计，旨在帮助学习者全面提升医疗英语水平，为他们在未来的医疗工作中有效沟通和应对挑战打下坚实的基础。

四、教材资源

为方便教师教学，帮助学习者自学，本教材有以下配套教学资源：

1. 通过搜索网站以及扫描书中二维码，学习者可以获取与教材相关的微课视频、视听练习视频以及课文和单词的音频资源。

2. PPT 课件与纸质教材无缝衔接，另有课后拓展、答案解析等材料供师生参考和系统学习。

五、编写团队

　　本教材得到了浙江省德育教材研究基地的项目资助，在此深表感谢！本教材由嘉兴大学吴嫣斐、苏娜担任主编，浙江中医药大学袁芳、吴素芳、谢苑苑担任副主编，参加编写的人员还有浙江中医药大学徐宁骏、宓芬芳、朱莹莹和嘉兴大学附属医院王宇。编者们在编写过程中参考、借鉴了国内外出版的相关书籍、论文和相关网站，在此一并致谢。

　　本教材集中了全体编者的智慧和心血，但因编者水平和经验有限，书中难免有不足之处，恳请读者不吝赐教，批评指正。

编写团队

Contents

Contents

Unit 1
Disease Prevention

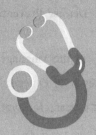

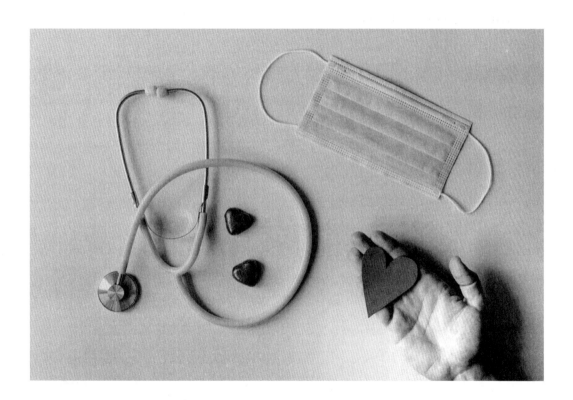

Over the past two decades, several high-impact pathogens have emerged or re-emerged. This trend of the increasing prevalence of pandemics is projected to continue, driven predominantly by urbanization, climate change, environmental degradation, and persistent social and economic inequality as well as the mass globalization of trade and travel. For any outbreak response system to be effective, it needs to be trusted, valued, and ultimately used by communities. That means reaching people where

Lead in

they are, in the language they speak, and aware of the culture, beliefs, and practices with which they live. One of the best ways to save lives is to invest in lasting health infrastructure, 365 days a year, for everyone, especially the most vulnerable among us.

This unit is mainly to achieve the following objectives:

1) Understand the prevention of disease focusing on some specific measures;

2) Identify words, phrases and sentence patterns related to the topic;

3) Make a poster by using the terminologies and medical information in this unit;

4) Learn the spirit of dedication.

Part I　View the Medical World

Watch a video about Ebola and choose the right answer.①

1. In 2013, how long did it take people to discover that Ebola was to blame for the death of a little boy in Guinea?

    A. Two months.   B. Four months.

    C. Two days.   D. Four days.

2. How many people were infected during the Ebola epidemic that began in 2013?

    A. Over 28,000.   B. Nearly 28,000.

    C. Over 11,000.   D. Nearly 11,000.

3. In 2021, Ebola was first transmitted to some people _____.

    A. in a hospital   B. in a church

    C. at a funeral   D. at a market

4. In 2021, what did people do to stop the spread of Ebola, except _____.

    A. activating emergency operations centers

    B. figuring out exactly who was exposed and when

    C. screening travelers

    D. building more hospitals

5. Which of the following statements is not an evidence that the 2021 outbreak brought less harm to people?

    A. Fewer people were infected.

    B. Fewer people died.

    C. Less money was spent controlling the outbreak.

    D. Fewer people did prevention work.

---

①　视频详见网站:https://pan-yz.cldisk.com/external/m/file/1055117140321103872。

Words and Phrases

Ebola /iˈbəulə/ *n.* 埃博拉(病毒)

Guinea /ˈgɪni/ *n.* 几内亚

devastating /ˈdevəsteɪtɪŋ/ *adj.* 毁灭性的

mushroom /ˈmʌʃrʊm/ *v.* 迅速增长

contract /ˈkɒntrækt/ *v.* 感染(疾病)；得(病)

contact tracer /ˈkɒntækt ˈtreɪsə(r)/ 接触者追踪人员

screening /ˈskriːnɪŋ/ *n.* 筛查

vaccine /ˈvæksiːn/ *n.* 疫苗

overhaul /ˌəuvəˈhɔːl/ *v.* 全面改革(制度、方法等)

spin up /spɪn ʌp/ 快速增长

pale /peɪl/ *v.* 显得逊色

Part II　Read to Explore Medical Knowledge

Text A

Pre-reading Questions:

1. Do you think wearing mask is an effective way to protect people from respiratory viral infections?

2. Besides wearing mask, can you think of other ways to protect people from infectious diseases?

Implementing a Comprehensive Strategy to Prevent Respiratory Viral Infections in Patients

Text A

1. A highly symbolic turning point in the SARS-CoV-2 pandemic has been reached with the lifting of the public health emergency in the U.S. The virus upended lives, changed health care drastically, and killed millions of people around the world at the height of the pandemic. The implementation of universal masking was a well publicized shift in health care, with the goal of lowering the SARS-CoV-2 transmission rate in health care facilities by the use of source control and exposure protection for all individuals present. However, now that the public health emergency has passed, many American health care facilities are reverting to a policy of requiring masking in limited situations, such as when attending to patients with potentially contagious respiratory infections, rather than universally.

2. Ceasing the use of masks outside of health care settings is justifiable. The morbidity and mortality linked to SARS-CoV-2 have significantly decreased due to the combination of immunity obtained from vaccination and infections, together with the widespread availability of rapid diagnostics and effective therapies. Since most people have long

handled influenza and other respiratory viruses without feeling compelled to mask, the majority of SARS-CoV-2 infections are currently no more severe than those infections.

3. However, there are two specific reasons why this framing is not widely applicable to health care facilities. To begin with, there are distinct differences between individuals who are hospitalized and those who are not. Hospitals aggregate some of the most vulnerable people in society when they are at heightened vulnerability. Vaccines and treatments for SARS-CoV-2 have decreased the occurrence and death rates linked to SARS-CoV-2 infections for most of the population. However, certain subgroups, such as older adults, individuals with immunocompromising conditions, and those with serious coexisting conditions like chronic lung disease or heart disease, still face an elevated risk of severe illness and death. A significant proportion of hospitalized patients at any one moment are comprised of individuals from these groups, many of whom also often utilize outpatient health care facilities.

4. Furthermore, it is important to note that nosocomial infections caused by respiratory viruses, excluding SARS-CoV-2, are frequently occurring but often not fully acknowledged. Additionally, the potential adverse health consequences linked to these viruses in susceptible patients are often underestimated. Instances of nosocomial transmissions and clusters of influenza, respiratory syncytial virus (RSV), human metapneumovirus, human parainfluenza virus, and other respiratory viruses occur with unexpected frequency. Viruses, rather than bacteria, may be the source of at least 20% of hospital-acquired pneumonia cases. Furthermore, the morbidity linked to respiratory infections goes beyond pneumonia. Viruses can potentially inflict significant damage by exacerbating patients' underlying conditions. Acute respiratory virus infections are known to be the triggers for obstructive lung disease flares, heart failure exacerbations, arrhythmias, ischemic events, neurologic events, and death. The influenza virus alone is linked to a maximum of 50,000 fatalities annually in the United States. On the other hand, measures meant to mitigate the harm caused by influenza, such as vaccination, are related with lower incidence of ischemia events, arrhythmias, heart failure exacerbations, and death in high-risk individuals.

5. Considering these factors, it is clear that masking is still a reasonable practice in health care settings. People with known and unknown respiratory virus infections can be contained by

wearing masks. Staff or visitors may not realize they are sick due to the mild and asymptomatic infections caused by respiratory viruses such as SARS-CoV-2, influenza, RSV, and others. However, it is important to note that even asymptomatic and presymptomatic persons can still transmit diseases to patients. In addition, "presenteeism" (going to work when sick) is popular, even though health care system executives have repeatedly asked symptomatic workers to stay home. Some health care facilities even reported that half of their SARS-CoV-2 infected employees continued to work despite experiencing symptoms during the peak of the outbreak. Medical professionals can prevent around 60% of nosocomial respiratory viral infections by using masks, according to studies conducted before and during the pandemic.

6. We understand that many health care professionals are eager to go back to pre-pandemic practices, that wearing a mask can be uncomfortable or impair communication, and that masking fatigue is common. Our proposed strategy involves connecting masking requirements judiciously to community viral transmission levels, workers' current activities, and individual patients' risk of severe sickness. This way, masking requirements can be applied prudently.

7. The transmission of respiratory viruses in the population is highly correlated with the prevalence of hospital-acquired respiratory viral infections. A higher viral infection rate in the population increases the likelihood that a health care provider, visitor, or patient may contract the virus and spread it to another patient. Therefore, health care facilities should think about calibrating masking strategies based on the transmission levels in the population. Rates of influenza-like illness or visits to the emergency department for influenza, RSV, and COVID-19 are examples of the kinds of surveillance metrics suggested by the Centers for Disease Control and Prevention that hospitals can use to initiate masking procedures. A further approach would be for facilities to anticipate when respiratory virus activity is likely to be highest and implement masking policies accordingly. Although this technique wouldn't be able to account for every time when respiratory viruses are circulating, it could be a fair compromise that protects patients more during peak dangers and less during low ones, lessening the imposition on health care personnel. As an added bonus, facilities would have an easier time communicating and preparing for the annual masking requirement if it were implemented during predetermined months rather than at random

intervals throughout the year in response to community transmission rates exceeding specific thresholds.

8. Likewise, not every situation calls for a mask at a health care facility. Due to the moral imperative to safeguard patients from nosocomial diseases, it is vital that all personnel and visitors wear masks whenever they come into contact with patients. Staff members are constantly exposed to respiratory viruses regardless of the facility's masking policy, since most of them no longer wear masks while they aren't at work. Therefore, there is less of a need to force them to mask outside of patient care. Again, there would be a happy medium between patient safety and employee burden if employees could choose to forgo masking when they were not directly involved with patients.

9. We maintain that clinical encounters involving patients at especially high risk for poor outcomes from respiratory viral infections should nonetheless require masking all year round, even if health care facilities choose to connect masking requirements to community transmission rates. Patients undergoing hematopoietic stem-cell transplantation, anti-CD20 agents, or organ transplantation (heart, lung, etc.) are examples of those with severe immunosuppression. Some respiratory viruses remain active all year, so even if these people have a reduced risk of infection when community transmission rates are low, it is never zero. Despite a low absolute risk, preventative measures are warranted due to the increased risk of severe disease in this population when a respiratory virus infection is present. The same goes for these patients; they should be reminded to always wear masks while they are in potentially dangerous environments.

10. Countless new details regarding respiratory virus morbidity, nosocomial transmission, and patient protection measures have emerged in the last three years from the fields of medicine and public health. In light of recent developments in the SARS-CoV-2 pandemic, it is reasonable to ease off on the need that everyone wear a mask while they are not in a health care setting, even at times when the transmission rate is low in the general population. Still, we think it's a poor decision to turn a blind eye to the fact that SARS-CoV-2 is still a danger to some individuals or that numerous other respiratory viruses are just as dangerous. Health care facilities should reimagine their current approach to masking as a means of protecting patients from SARS-CoV-2 and other nosocomial respiratory viral infections. By implementing a system that applies masks to all patients during periods of high viral activity and to the most susceptible individuals all year round, they can better safeguard their

patients from the full spectrum of nosocomial respiratory viral infections.

✍ New Words and Expressions

New Words and
Expressions

SARS-CoV-2 /ˌsɑːz kəʊˌviːˈtuː/ Severe Acute Respiratory Syndrome-Coronavirus 2：the strain of a coronavirus that causes COVID-19. First identified in 2019，it subsequently set off a global pandemic. 严重急性呼吸综合征冠状病毒 2 型

pandemic /pænˈdemɪk/ n. a disease that spreads over a whole country or the whole world（全国或全球性）流行病；大流行病

upend /ʌpˈend/ v. to turn sb. /sth. upside down 翻倒；倒放；使颠倒

transmission /trænzˈmɪʃn/ n. the act or process of passing sth. from one person, place or thing to another 传送；传递；传达；传播；传染

health care facility A health care facility is a location where medical and health services are provided to diagnose, treat, and manage illnesses, injuries, and other health conditions. 医疗机构

exposure /ɪkˈspəʊʒə(r)/ n. the fact or state of being exposed 接触；暴露

revert /rɪˈvɜːt/ v. to return to a former habit, practice, belief, condition, etc. 恢复；回复（到以前的状态、制度或行为）

contagious /kənˈteɪdʒəs/ adj. capable of being transmitted by bodily contact with an infected person or object 接触传染的

respiratory /rəˈspɪrətri/ adj. connected with breathing 呼吸的

infection /ɪnˈfekʃn/ n. the act or process of causing or getting a disease 传染；感染

morbidity /mɔːˈbɪdəti/ n. the proportion of sickness or of a specific disease in a geographical locality 发病率

mortality /mɔːˈtæləti/ n. the number of deaths in a particular situation or period of time 死亡数量；死亡率

immunity /ɪˈmjuːnəti/ n. the body's ability to avoid or not be affected by infection and disease 免疫力

vaccination /ˌvæksɪˈneɪʃən/ n. the act of vaccinating 接种疫苗

diagnostics /ˌdaɪəgˈnɒstɪkz/ *n.* the practice or methods of diagnosis (= finding out what is wrong with a person who is ill/sick) 诊断；诊断法

influenza /ˌɪnfluˈenzə/ *n.* an acute febrile highly contagious viral disease 流行性感冒

compel /kəmˈpel/ *v.* to force sb. to do sth. ; to make sth. necessary 强迫；迫使；使必须

framing /ˈfreɪmɪŋ/ *n.* formulation of the plans and important details 构架；框架；构架系统

aggregate /ˈægrɪgət/ *v.* to put together different items, amounts, etc. into a single group or total 总计；汇集

vulnerable /ˈvʌlnərəbl/ *adj.* weak and easily hurt physically or emotionally (身体上或感情上)脆弱的；易受……伤害的

heightened /ˈhaɪtənd/ *adj.* stronger or more vigorous 加强的；加剧的

subgroup /ˈsʌbgruːp/ *n.* a smaller group made up of members of a larger group 小组；(团体中的)部分

immunocompromising /ˌɪmjuːnəʊˈkɒmprəmaɪzɪŋ/ *adj.* having the immune system impaired or weakened 免疫功能受损的

coexisting /ˌkəʊɪgˈzɪstɪŋ/ *adj.* existing at the same time 共存的

chronic /ˈkrɒnɪk/ *adj.* lasting for a long time；difficult to cure or get rid of 长期的；慢性的；难以治愈(或根除)的

elevate /ˈelɪveɪt/ *v.* to make the level of sth. increase 提高；使升高

outpatient /ˈaʊtpeɪʃnt/ *n.* a person who goes to a hospital for treatment but does not stay there 门诊病人

nosocomial /ˌnɒsəˈkəʊmɪəl/ *adj.* taking place or originating in a hospital 医院的

underestimate /ˌʌndərˈestɪmeɪt/ *v.* to make too low an estimate of the quantity, degree, or worth of 低估；对……估计不足

adverse /ˈædvɜːs/ *adj.* negative and unpleasant；not likely to produce a good result 不利的；有害的；反面的

cluster /ˈklʌstə(r)/ *n.* a number of things of the same kind, growing or held together；a bunch 团；群；簇

syncytial /sɪnˈsɪʃɪəl/ *adj.* related to the merging of individual cells into a larger, unified structure that functions collectively 合胞体的

metapneumovirus /ˈmetənjuːmuːˈvaɪrəs/ *n.* a family of viruses that infect the respiratory tract and cause respiratory illness in humans and animals 偏肺病毒

parainfluenza /ˌpærəɪnfluˈenzə/ *n.* a group of viruses that infect the respiratory tract and cause similar symptoms to those of influenza, but are less severe 副流感

pneumonia /njuːˈməʊniə/ *n.* a serious illness affecting one or both lungs that makes breathing difficult 肺炎

exacerbate /ɪɡˈzæsəbeɪt/ *v.* to make sth. worse, especially a disease or problem 使恶化；使加剧；使加重

underlying /ˌʌndəˈlaɪɪŋ/ *adj.* important in a situation but not always easily noticed or stated clearly 根本的；潜在的；隐含的

trigger /ˈtrɪɡə(r)/ *n.* something that is the cause of a particular reaction or development, especially a bad one (尤指引发不良反应或发展的)起因；诱因

obstructive /əbˈstrʌktɪv/ *adj.* connected with a passage, tube, etc. in your body that has become blocked 梗阻的；阻塞的；栓塞的

flare /fleə(r)/ *n.* a sudden recurrence or worsening of symptoms (疾病、伤势)突然复发；突然恶化

arrhythmia /əˈrɪðmɪə/ *n.* any disturbance in the rhythm of the heartbeat 心律失常；心律不齐

ischemic /ɪsˈkiːmɪk/ *adj.* relating to or affected by ischemia 缺血性的

neurologic /njʊərəʊˈlɒdʒɪk/ *adj.* of or relating to or used in or practicing neurology 神经病学的

mitigate /ˈmɪtɪɡeɪt/ *v.* to make sth. less harmful, serious, etc. 减轻；缓和

asymptomatic /ˌeɪsɪmptəˈmætɪk/ *adj.* having no symptoms of illness or disease 无临床症状的

presymptomatic /priːsɪmptəˈmætɪk/ *adj.* of or relating to the early phases of a disease when accurate diagnosis is not possible because symptoms of the disease have not yet appeared 症状发生前的

presenteeism /ˌprezn̩ˈtiːɪzəm/ *n.* the practice of spending more time at your work than you need to according to your contract 超时工作

impair /ɪmˈpeə(r)/ *v.* to damage sth. or make sth. worse 损害；削弱

judiciously /dʒuˈdɪʃəslɪ/ adv. careful and sensible；showing good judgement 审慎而明智地；明断地；有见地地

calibrate /ˈkælɪbreɪt/ v. to measure precisely 精确测量；准确估量

surveillance /sɜːˈveɪləns/ n. close observation of a person or group 监督；管制

metrics /ˈmetrɪks/ n. standard of measurement 指标；量度

circulate /ˈsɜːkjəleɪt/ v. to cause to pass from place to place，person to person 传播

imposition /ˌɪmpəˈzɪʃn/ n. an unfair or unreasonable thing that sb. expects or asks you to do 不公平(或不合理)的要求

threshold /ˈθreʃhəʊld/ n. the level at which sth. starts to happen or have an effect 阈；界；起始点

imperative /ɪmˈperətɪv/ n. a thing that is very important and needs immediate attention or action 重要紧急的事；必要的事

forgo /fɔːˈɡəʊ/ v. to decide not to have or do sth. that you would like to have or do 放弃，弃绝(想做的事或想得之物)

hematopoietic /ˌhemətəʊpɔɪˈetɪk/ adj. pertaining to the formation of blood or blood cells 造血的；生血的

agent /ˈeɪdʒənt/ n. a chemical or a substance that produces an effect or a change or is used for a particular purpose 药剂；药物

immunosuppression /ˌɪmjunəʊsəˈpreʃn/ n. the act of stopping the body from reacting against antigens，for example in order to prevent the body from rejecting a new organ 免疫抑制

warranted /ˈwɒrəntɪd/ adj. backed or covered by a warranty or guarantee 担保的；保证的

reimagine /riːɪˈmædʒɪn/ v. to think about or consider in a new and creative way 重新构想

▤ Notes

1. respiratory syncytial virus（RSV）：Respiratory syncytial virus, or RSV, is a common respiratory virus that usually causes mild, cold-like symptoms. Most people recover in a week

or two, but RSV can be serious, especially for infants and older adults. RSV is the most common cause of bronchiolitis (inflammation of the small airways in the lung) and pneumonia (infection of the lungs) in children younger than 1 year of age.

呼吸道合胞病毒(RSV)是一种常见的呼吸道病毒，通常会引起轻微的感冒样症状。大多数人在一两周内康复，但呼吸道合胞病毒可能很严重，尤其是对婴儿和老年人来说。呼吸道合胞病毒是 1 岁以下儿童细支气管炎(肺部小气道炎症)和肺炎(肺部感染)的最常见原因。

2. human metapneumovirus：Human metapneumovirus (HMPV) can cause upper and lower respiratory disease in people of all ages, especially among young children, older adults, and people with weakened immune systems. It was Discovered in 2001. Symptoms commonly associated with HMPV include cough, fever, nasal congestion, and shortness of breath. Clinical symptoms of HMPV infection may progress to bronchitis or pneumonia.

人偏肺病毒(HMPV)可在所有年龄段的人中引起上下呼吸道疾病，尤其是在幼儿、老年人和免疫系统较弱的人中。HMPV 于 2001 年被发现。常见症状包括咳嗽、发热、鼻塞和呼吸急促。HMPV 感染在临床上可能发展为支气管炎或肺炎。

3. human parainfluenza virus：Human parainfluenza viruses (HPIVs) commonly cause respiratory infections in infants and young children. Patients usually recover on their own. However, HPIVs can also cause more severe illness, such as croup or pneumonia. Flu vaccine will not protect you against HPIVs infections. HPIVs usually spread by direct contact with infectious droplets or by airborne spread when an infected person breathes, coughs, or sneezes.

人副流感病毒(HPIVs)通常会导致婴幼儿呼吸道感染。患者通常自行康复。然而，HPIVs 也可能导致更严重的疾病，如哮吼或肺炎。流感疫苗不能使人免受 HPIVs 感染。HPIVs 通常通过直接接触传染性飞沫传播，或通过感染者呼吸、咳嗽或打喷嚏时的空气传播。

4. Centers for Disease Control and Prevention (CDC)：美国疾病控制与预防中心

5. hematopoietic stem-cell transplantation：Hematopoietic stem-cell transplantation is a procedure used to treat certain types of blood cancer and immune disorders. Hematopoietic stem cells produce red blood cells, white blood cells, and platelets, primarily in the bone marrow. The stem cells can be harvested from the peripheral blood, bone marrow, or newborn umbilical blood. The recipient undergoes a conditioning regimen to clear their bone marrow of

hematopoietic stem cells. Then they receive the transplant as an infusion. After the transplant, the cells migrate to the bone marrow and produce new blood cells and immune cells.

　　造血干细胞移植是一种用于治疗某些类型血液癌症和免疫疾病的治疗手段。造血干细胞主要在骨髓中产生红细胞、白细胞和血小板。干细胞可以从外周血、骨髓或新生儿脐带血中获得。接受者接受调理方案以清除其骨髓中的造血干细胞。然后他们以输液的方式接受移植。移植后，细胞迁移到骨髓，产生新的血细胞和免疫细胞。

After Reading Activities

Reading Comprehension

I. Answer the following questions.

1. Why is discontinuing masking outside of health care contexts understandable?

2. Why does masking in health care facilities continue to make sense?

3. What can reduce nosocomial respiratory viral infections by approximately 60% according to the studies?

4. What can people do to apply masking requirements wisely?

5. What kind of patients should be advised to wear masks themselves in higher-risk situations year-round?

II. Work in groups to complete the following chart according to the structure of the text.

The current situation: (paras. 1-2)

　　During the height of the pandemic, one of the most visible changes in health care was _____, a measure designed to reduce SARS-CoV-2 transmission in health care facilities by the use of _____ and _____ to everyone in the facility. With the end of the public health emergency, however, many health care centers in the United States are now stopping universal masking. _____ outside of health care settings is justifiable.

The necessities of masking application in health care facilities: (paras. 3-5)

1. Most _____ people in society are gathered in health care facilities. (para. 3)

2. _____ caused by respiratory viruses other than SARS-CoV-2 are common and underestimated. (para. 4)

3. People with _____ respiratory virus infections can be contained by wearing masks. (para. 5)

Solutions to apply masking requirements judiciously: (paras. 6-9)

1. We acknowledge that there is widespread _____ among health care workers. (para. 6)

2. The Centers for Disease Control and Prevention has suggested _____ that hospitals can use to trigger masking requirements. The strategy of requiring masking during _____ each year would also involve simpler communication and planning for facilities. (para. 7)

3. _____ calls for a mask at a health care facility. (para. 8)

4. Health care facilities should still require _____ for clinical interactions involving patients at particularly high risk for _____ from respiratory viral infections. (para. 9)

Conclusion: (para. 10)

Rather than abandoning universal masking for protection against SARS-CoV-2, health care facilities should _____ as a means of protecting patients from SARS-CoV-2 and other nosocomial respiratory viral infections.

Words and Phrases

✅ I. Translate the following medical terms into Chinese or English.

1. respiratory viral infection   _____

2. health care facility   _____

3. immunocompromising condition   _____

4. obstructive lung disease   _____

5. 无症状感染   _____

6. 监控指标   _____

7. 社区传播   _____

8. 公共卫生   _____

✅ II. Fill in the blanks with the words or phrases given below. Change the form if necessary.

exposure	aggregate	adverse	circulate	trigger

1. Eighty percent of parents knew at least one of the _____ that worsened their children's asthma.

2. The players' scores will be _____ by the average rank from fan, player and media votes, and the fan vote will be the tiebreaker.

3. Analysis of laboratory samples showed that the new virus had never before _____ in humans.

4. The _____ effects of the drug are too severe to allow it to be marketed.

5. In other words, it's the adolescent confusion and the _____ to the real world that make youthful days so special.

Sentence Translation

Translate the following sentences into Chinese or English.

1. The morbidity and mortality linked to SARS-CoV-2 have significantly decreased due to the combination of immunity obtained from vaccination and infections, together with the widespread availability of rapid diagnostics and effective therapies.

_____

_____

2. Instances of nosocomial transmissions and clusters of influenza, respiratory syncytial virus (RSV), human metapneumovirus, parainfluenza virus, and other respiratory viruses occur with unexpected frequency.

_____

_____

3. Staff members are constantly exposed to respiratory viruses regardless of the facility's masking policy, since most of them no longer wear masks while they aren't at work. Therefore, there is less of a need to force them to mask outside of patient care.

_____

4. 如果人群中病毒感染率较高，医疗服务提供者、访客或患者感染病毒并将病毒传播给其他患者的可能性就会增加。

_____

_____

_____

5. 通过实施在病毒高发期让所有病人佩戴口罩，以及全年让最易感人群佩戴口罩的体系，他们可以更好地保护患者免受各种医院呼吸道病毒感染。

_____

_____

_____

Text B

Pre-reading Questions:

1. Do you know any diseases that threaten the public health?

2. Are there any effective ways that governments or individuals can take to improve the public health?

The Reasons for the Emergence of Global Health as the New Public Health

Text B

1. Between early May and July 23, the number of monkeypox cases increased dramatically to over 16,000 in 75 countries, many of which had not previously experienced the virus. On July 23, the World Health Organization called the epidemic a "public health emergency of international concern." As of August 17, there were 32,000 confirmed cases; the first deaths from monkeypox outside of Africa occurred in Brazil, India, and Spain; and the infection rate showed no indications of decreasing as nations battled to control the new virus.

2. According to Dr. Ingrid Katz, associate faculty director of the Harvard Global Health Institute, in today's society, an infectious disease has the ability to rapidly travel throughout the globe within a few hours. Due to the widespread use of air travel and the interconnectedness of global business and economy, any impact on one country has repercussions for other nations, be it a viral outbreak or a decline in children immunization rates. No nation is an island when it comes to health.

3. To understand how professionals are prioritizing global concerns, one must grasp that public health extends far beyond national boundaries. For international health agencies, these will be among the most pressing concerns in the years ahead.

Identifying and Curtailing the Impact of Pandemics

4. An international agreement to enhance global pandemic prevention, preparedness, and response is currently being drafted by the World Health Assembly, the decision-making

body of the World Health Organization. David Ross, CEO and president of the Task Force for Global Health in Atlanta, says that if nations can come to an agreement, international pandemic threat detection and response treaties would allow every country to have a trained workforce of field epidemiologists—basically, international disease detectives—and to bolster disease surveillance systems and laboratory and diagnostic capabilities.

5. One of the thorny issues is determining the most efficient approach, potentially involving incentives, to motivate governments to promptly report outbreaks. "Even slight delays in reporting can have a significant impact on the extent to which an infectious disease spreads. Currently, there are disincentives to reporting, such as travel bans, which negatively affect the economies of countries," states Ross.

6. Simultaneously, the U.S. Centers for Disease Control and Prevention is broadening its efforts worldwide to enhance the identification, documentation, and reaction to outbreaks. An article by Dr. Kevin Cain, primary deputy director of the CDC's Center for Global Health, states that the organization has offices in over 50 nations. In these locations, CDC scientists and local staff collaborate with the host nation's health ministries to enhance these abilities. These efforts were successful during the COVID-19 pandemic. The areas where we put our money were much better able to identify epidemics and report them immediately. Members of our global personnel, who are typically naturalized citizens, performed heroic deeds. They assisted their respective health ministries in responding to the crisis when we were unable to send a large number of personnel.

Vaccine Development and Distribution

7. According to Cain, "vaccines don't do any good sitting in vials," but they did learn during the COVID-19 pandemic that even newly discovered diseases may be made avoidable by vaccines rather rapidly. "It is critical that we improve distribution so that we can get shots into arms." In low-income nations, just 20% of the population has gotten the COVID-19 vaccine, while in ten states in the U.S., the entire immunization rate is lower than 57%. Viruses still have ample opportunity to spread and mutate with huge populations of people who have not gotten the vaccine, either because they cannot afford it or because they have been misled about the benefits. This is one of the factors contributing to the ongoing emergence of novel variants of COVID-19. Cain explains that their goal is to assist nations

in better conveying the advantages of vaccines through communication.

8. Aiding nations in developing their own capacity to produce and disperse vaccines is one possible way to streamline vaccine distribution, according to Katz. She argues that while some regions like Africa, Brazil, and India are taking the lead, the movement should be far more widespread. We have neglected vaccines as a public benefit in favor of treating them like a commodity for far too long. To get everyone vaccinated, businesses must be willing to waive patents and share data and supplies.

9. Simultaneously, experts in global health have sounded the alarm on the urgency of intensifying efforts in childhood vaccines. The World Health Organization (WHO) and the United Nations International Children's Emergency Fund (UNICEF) have reported a significant and prolonged decrease in children immunizations, marking the most substantial reduction in the past three decades. In 2021, around 25 million children did not receive one or more doses of the vaccine for diphtheria, tetanus, and pertussis. "The reason for this is COVID-19, which has significantly depleted the health workforce," explains Stephen Morrison, the head of the Global Health Policy Center at the Center for Strategic & International Studies. Currently, the priority is learning to walk and chew gum at the same time by adapting to and addressing pandemics, while also revitalizing and enhancing the significant progress achieved in the field of pediatric immunizations over the past three decades. Unless we increase vaccination rates to the necessary level, we can see an uptick in cases and fatalities from illnesses that were previously under control.

10. Currently, the eradication of polio has been successful in most nations, with the exception of Pakistan and Afghanistan. Following the suspension of the immunization campaign by the Global Polio Eradication Initiative in 2020, a polio epidemic occurred in Malawi in late 2021. The United Kingdom saw its inaugural epidemic in 40 years in June 2022. In July, a guy in New York who had not had a vaccination was diagnosed with the condition and experienced paralysis. The virus has subsequently been identified in sewage in New York City and other parts of the state.

Tackling Food Insecurity and Alleviating Poverty

11. There was a 150 million increase in the number of hungry people since the epidemic began in 2020, reaching 828 million, according to the FAO's State of Food Security and

Nutrition in the World 2022 report. "Hunger is a huge issue, and it's getting bigger every day," remarks Emily Janoch, senior director of learning at CARE, an international humanitarian organization fighting world hunger and poverty. "While there are pockets of hungry people in every nation, the pandemic, the conflict in Ukraine, and the environmental catastrophe have made their problems worse." For example, several countries are experiencing food insecurity since they depend on imports of grain, cooking oil, and fertilizer from Russia and Ukraine. This includes Ethiopia, Afghanistan, Yemen, and Somalia.

12. It is not just emotionally distressing; it is also potentially hazardous. Malnourished individuals are at a higher risk of contracting infectious diseases and have reduced capacity to contribute to the economy. This situation destabilizes a country's workforce and poses a threat to its economic stability. Consequently, it undermines their capacity to carry out efficient public health campaigns, ranging from nutrition programs to the provision of vaccines.

13. The United States pledged as much as 11 billion dollars to combat global malnutrition at the Tokyo Nutrition for Growth Summit in 2021. In addition, it initiated the Global Nutrition Coordination Plan, a set of six objectives that aim to improve people's diets by making sure they get enough micronutrients, preventing and managing childhood wasting, and supporting women's nutrition before, during, and after pregnancy.

14. It is crucial to support farmers, particularly women farmers, by investing in them. They supply half of the world's agricultural labor, yet they are frequently denied land ownership, decision-making authority, and adequate equipment, seeds, and fertilizer. The FAO found that if women in developing nations had equal access to agricultural resources, production on women's farms might increase by 20 to 30 percent.

Boosting Medical Treatment and Technological Capabilities

15. Artificial intelligence (AI) has the potential to fill the most pressing knowledge and judgment gaps, which contribute to the 8.4 million annual deaths and $1.6 trillion in lost productivity caused by subpar health care in low-and middle-income nations, according to Katz.

16. According to Katz, in order to fully achieve the potential of AI in the realm of global

health, it is necessary to have dependable and high-caliber data. This data is used to train AI systems to make optimal decisions and to enable them to oversee and handle the always evolving technology. "When utilized efficiently, artificial intelligence has the capacity to completely transform the field of global health and health care."

17. Health care providers, particularly in more remote locations, frequently work independently, without access to specialists or pharmacists, in nations with some of the world's lowest doctor-to-population ratios, such as Ethiopia or Nigeria. As a result of having to cater to so many different types of patients, the quality of care they deliver suffers. Artificial intelligence systems can assist doctors with patient diagnoses and treatment plan selection, perhaps reducing the overuse of antibiotics. In extreme circumstances, AI could even replace a human doctor.

New Words and Expressions

New Words and Expressions

monkeypox / ˈmʌŋkiːpɒks/ *n.* a viral zoonotic infection caused by the monkeypox virus 猴痘

associate /əˈsəʊsieɪt, əˈsəʊʃieɪt/ *adj.* of a lower rank, having fewer rights in a particular profession or organization (常用于头衔) 非正式的; 准的; 副的

interconnectedness /ˌɪntəkəˈnektɪdnəs/ *n.* the quality or condition of being interconnected 相互联系; 相互关联

repercussion /ˌriːpəˈkʌʃn/ *n.* an indirect and usually bad result of an action or event that may happen some time afterwards (间接的) 影响; 反响; 恶果

prioritize /praɪˈɒrətaɪz/ *v.* to put tasks, problems, etc. in order of importance, so that you can deal with the most important first 按重要性排列; 划分优先顺序

curtail /kɜːˈteɪl/ *v.* to limit sth. or make it last for a shorter time 限制; 缩短; 减缩

epidemiologist /ˌepɪˌdiːmɪ ˈɒlədʒɪst/ *n.* a medical scientist who studies the transmission and control of epidemic diseases 流行病学家

bolster /ˈbəʊlstə(r)/ *v.* to improve sth. or make it stronger 改善; 加强

thorny /ˈθɔːni/ *adj.* causing difficulty or disagreement 棘手的; 麻烦的; 引起争议的

incentive /ɪnˈsentɪv/ *n.* something that encourages you to do sth. 激励; 刺激; 鼓励

distribution /dɪˈstrɪbjuːʃn/ *n.* the act of giving or delivering sth to a number of people 分发；分送

vial /ˈvaɪəl/ *n.* a small bottle that contains a drug（装香水、药物等的）小瓶

ample /ˈæmpl/ *adj.* enough or more than enough 足够的；丰裕的

mutate /mjuːˈteɪt/ *v.* to develop or make sth. develop a new form or structure, because of a genetic change（使）变异；突变

variant /ˈveəriənt/ *n.* a thing that is a slightly different form or type of sth. else 变种；变体；变形

waive /weɪv/ *v.* to choose not to demand sth. in a particular case, even though you have a legal or official right to do so 放弃（权利、要求等）

patent /ˈpeɪtnt, ˈpætnt/ *n.* an official right to be the only person to make, use or sell a product or an invention; a document that proves this 专利权；专利证书

sound /saʊnd/ *v.* to give a signal such as a warning by making a sound 鸣警报；拉响警报；发出警报

dose /dəʊs/ *n.* an amount of a medicine or a drug that is taken once, or regularly over a period of time（药的）一剂；一服

diphtheria /dɪfˈθɪəriə/ *n.* a highly contagious bacterial infection which affects the respiratory tract, but can also affect the skin, nose, throat, and other parts of the body 白喉

tetanus /ˈtetənəs/ *n.* a serious and potentially life-threatening bacterial infection which affects the nervous system and is characterized by muscle stiffness 破伤风

pertussis /pəˈtʌsɪs/ *n.* a highly contagious respiratory disease characterized by severe, persistent coughing fits that can make it hard for an infected person to breathe 百日咳

walk and chew gum at the same time often used metaphorically to describe someone who can perform multiple tasks simultaneously without any difficulty 双管齐下

address /əˈdres/ *v.* to think about a problem or a situation and decide how you are going to deal with it 设法解决；处理；对付

revitalize /ˌriːˈvaɪtəlaɪz/ *v.* to make sth. stronger, more active or healthier 使更强壮；使恢复生机(或健康)

uptick /ˈʌptɪk/ *n.* a small increase 小幅增加

eradication /ɪˌrædɪkeɪʃn/ *n.* the complete destruction of sth., especially sth. bad 根除；消灭；杜绝

polio /ˈpəʊliəʊ/ *n.* a highly infectious viral disease that primarily affects young children and can lead to paralysis or even death in severe cases 脊髓灰质炎（等于 poliomyelitis）

immunization /ˌɪmjʊnaɪˈzeɪʃn/ *n.* the act of making someone or something immune or the state of being immune 免疫

initiative /ɪˈnɪʃətɪv/ *n.* a new plan for dealing with a particular problem or for achieving a particular purpose 倡议；新方案

paralysis /pəˈræləsɪs/ *n.* a loss of control of, and sometimes feeling in, part or most of the body, caused by disease or an injury to the nerves 麻痹；瘫痪

pockets of commonly used to describe small, localized areas or groups within a larger context that differ significantly from the surrounding environment in terms of characteristics, conditions, or behavior 一些

malnourished /ˌmælˈnʌrɪʃt/ *adj.* in bad health because of a lack of food or a lack of the right type of food 营养不良的

destabilize /ˌdiːˈsteɪbəlaɪz/ *v.* to make a system, country, government, etc. become less firmly established or successful 使（制度、国家、政府等）动摇；使不安定；使不稳定

undermine /ˌʌndəˈmaɪn/ *v.* to make sth., especially sb.'s confidence or authority, gradually weaker or less effective 逐渐削弱（信心、权威等）；使逐步减少效力

malnutrition /ˌmælnjuːˈtrɪʃn/ *n.* a poor condition of health caused by a lack of food or a lack of the right type of food 营养不良

micronutrient /ˌmaikrəʊˈnjuːtriənt/ *n.* a substance needed only in small amounts for normal body function (e.g. vitamins or minerals) 微量营养素

wasting /ˈweɪstɪŋ/ *n.* any general reduction in vitality and strength of body and mind resulting from a debilitating chronic disease 消瘦

pregnancy /ˈpregnənsi/ *n.* the state of being pregnant 怀孕；妊娠；孕期

realm /relm/ *n.* an area of activity, interest, or knowledge 领域；场所

oversee /ˌəʊvəˈsiː/ *v.* to watch sb./sth. and make sure that a job or an activity is done correctly 监督；监视

pharmacist /ˈfɑːməsɪst/ *n.* a person whose job is to prepare medicines and sell or give them to the public in a shop/store or in a hospital 药剂师

ratio /ˈreɪʃiəʊ/ *n.* the relationship in quantity, amount, or size between two or more things 比率；比例

antibiotics /ˌæntɪbaɪˈɑtɪks/ *n.* a substance, for example penicillin, that can destroy or prevent the growth of bacteria and cure infections 抗菌素；抗生素

Notes

1. monkeypox：A zoonotic disease especially of central and western Africa that is caused by a poxvirus (species Monkeypox virus of the genus Orthopoxvirus), that is transmitted in humans usually by direct contact with the infectious lesions or bodily fluids of an infected person or animal, and that causes initial symptoms including fever, headache, swollen lymph glands, myalgia, and fatigue followed by skin eruptions typically on the face, hands, feet, and mouth with lesions that eventually fill with fluid before sloughing off. The World Health Organization (WHO) announced on November 28, 2022 that it will begin using the name mpox to refer to this disease due to the stigmatizing nature of the original name.

一种人畜共患病，主要发生在非洲中部和西部，由痘病毒(猴痘病毒属)引起，通常通过直接接触感染者或动物的传染性皮损或体液传播给人类，最初症状包括发热、头痛、淋巴结肿大、肌痛和疲劳，随后出现皮肤糜烂，通常发生在面部、手部、足部和口腔，皮损最终充满液体，然后脱落。世界卫生组织(WHO)于 2022 年 11 月 28 日宣布，由于原名具有污名化性质，将开始使用 mpox 这一名称来指代该疾病。

2. Harvard Global Health Institute：哈佛全球健康研究所

3. World Health Assembly：The World Health Assembly is the decision-making body of WHO. The main functions of the World Health Assembly are to determine the policies of the Organization, appoint the Director-General, supervise financial policies, and review and approve the proposed programme budget. The World Health Assembly is held annually in Geneva, Switzerland.

世界卫生大会是世界卫生组织的决策机构。世界卫生大会的主要职能是确定本组织的政策、任命总干事、监督财务政策以及审查和批准拟议方案预算。世界卫生大会每年在瑞士日内瓦举行。

4. UNICEF：联合国儿童基金会（United Nations International Children's Emergency Fund）

5. diphtheria：An acute febrile contagious disease typically marked by the formation of a false membrane especially in the throat and caused by a gram-positive bacterium（Corynebacterium diphtheriae）that produces a toxin causing inflammation of the heart and nervous system.

白喉是一种急性发热性传染病，通常以形成假膜为特征，尤其是在喉咙，由革兰氏阳性细菌（白喉棒状杆菌）引起，该细菌产生毒素，引起心脏和神经系统炎症。

6. tetanus：Tetanus is an infection caused by bacteria called Clostridium tetani. When these bacteria enter the body, they produce a toxin that causes painful muscle contractions. Another name for tetanus is "lockjaw". It often causes a person's neck and jaw muscles to lock, making it hard to open the mouth or swallow.

破伤风是由一种叫作破伤风梭菌的细菌引起的感染。这些细菌进入人体后会产生一种毒素，导致肌肉收缩疼痛。破伤风的另一个名称是"lockjaw"。它通常会导致患者的颈部和下颌肌肉锁定，使其难以张口或吞咽。

7. pertussis：An infectious respiratory disease especially of children caused by a bacterium（Bordetella pertussis）and marked by a convulsive spasmodic cough sometimes followed by a crowing intake of breath.

百日咳是一种传染性呼吸道疾病，尤指由一种细菌（百日咳杆菌）引起的儿童呼吸道疾病，其特征是抽搐性痉挛性咳嗽，有时伴有急促的呼吸。

8. the Center for Strategic & International Studies：美国战略与国际研究中心

9. polio：Polio, or poliomyelitis, is a disabling and life-threatening disease caused by the poliovirus. The virus spreads from person to person and can infect a person's spinal cord, causing paralysis（can't move parts of the body）.

脊髓灰质炎是由脊髓灰质炎病毒引起的具有致残性和危及生命的疾病。这种病毒在人与人之间传播，并会感染人的脊髓，导致瘫痪（无法移动身体的某些部位）。

10. the Food and Agriculture Organization of the United Nations(FAO)：联合国粮食及农业组织

11. State of Food Security and Nutrition in the World 2022 report：2022 年《世界粮食安全和营养状况》报告

📄 After Reading Activities

Reading Comprehension

Decide whether the following statements are true (T) or false (F) according to the text.

_____ 1. Infectious disease only spreads fast and harms people in developing countries.

_____ 2. The World Health Assembly is working with the ministries of health of many countries to improve outbreak detection, reporting and response of infectious disease.

_____ 3. Viruses are more likely to spread and mutate because many people are unvaccinated.

_____ 4. Hunger destabilizes countries' economy and makes it harder to implement effective campaigns for vaccine distribution.

_____ 5. Reliable, high-quality data can help AI to improve the quality of health care.

Words and Phrases

Match each English phrase in Column A with its Chinese version in Column B.

Column A	Column B
1. disease surveillance system	A. 社会公益
2. diagnostic capability	B. 疫苗供应
3. Health Commission	C. 医疗服务人员
4. public benefit	D. 诊断能力
5. food insecurity	E. 治疗方案
6. provision of vaccines	F. 卫生部
7. health care provider	G. 粮食短缺
8. treatment plan	H. 疾病监测系统

Translation

长期以来，公共卫生的官员们一直在寻求一种预防疟疾（malaria）的疫苗，疟疾每年感染6亿人，造成40万人死亡，其中大部分是儿童。2021年，这方面取得了重大进展。在一项针对450名儿童的研究中，研究人员报告说，一种名为R21的新型疟疾疫苗的有效率为77%。不过，这项研究的样本群体相对较小，还需要更多的研究。包括牛津大学在内的一个国际团队的研究人员计划对最初的样本组进行更长时间的跟踪，并将在疟疾常年活跃的国家开展其他试验。

Critical Thinking

The Chinese government has made significant efforts to improve the public health. Please work in groups to have a discussion focusing on one policy enacted by the Chinese government aiming to guarantee the public health and how this policy works.

Part III   Apply Medical English

✅ A. Situational Dialogues in Different Clinical Departments

Dialogue

Internal Medicine(内科)

Influenza(流感)

Doctor: Good morning! Please take a seat. What seems to be the problem?

Patient: Good morning, doctor! I've got a splitting headache and felt pain in all my joints and muscles for two days. My temperature is about 38℃.

Doctor: OK, please tell me how it got started.

Patient: I had a running nose last week. But I thought it was just a common cold and it would be better soon. But now it is getting worse!

Doctor: You also sound a bit hoarse. Don't worry. Let me give you an examination. Open your mouth and say "ah".

Patient: Ah.

Doctor: Good. Now, let me exam your chest. Take a deep breath in and out. By the way, do you have a history of tuberculosis? Or have you ever had any chronic ailments of respiratory system?

Patient: No, definitely not.

Doctor: Look, your throat is inflamed. And your tongue is thickly coated. You have all the symptoms of influenza.

Patient: Is it serious, doctor?

Doctor: According to your general situation, it's not so serious. Take a good rest, drink more water and avoid greasy food. I will write you a prescription.

Patient: That's a relief. I'll do as you say. Thank you very much, doctor.

Words and Phrases

splitting headache /ˈsplɪtɪŋ ˈhedeɪk/ 头痛欲裂

running nose /ˈrʌnɪŋ nəʊz/ 流鼻涕

hoarse /hɔːs/ *adj.* 嘶哑的

tuberculosis /tjuːˌbɜːkjuˈləʊsɪs/ *n.* 肺结核

chronic ailment /ˈkrɒnɪk ˈeɪlmənt/ 慢性疾病

respiratory system /rəˈspɪrətri ˈsɪstəm/ 呼吸系统

inflamed /ɪnˈfleɪmd/ *adj.* 发炎的；红肿的

Notes

Internal medicine

Internal medicine is a specialty of clinical medicine. It is a broad field that includes diseases and conditions of the organs such as heart, lungs, kidneys, liver, pancreas and thyroid. Internal medicine doctors are responsible for managing diseases such as diabetes, high blood pressure, and high cholesterol.

Here are some most common internal medicine diseases.

Respiratory diseases

General internists, as well as those who choose pulmonary medicine as their sub-area, often help patients who are living with respiratory problems. They will provide these patients with a proper diagnosis, as well as provide them with any treatment or management services they need in order to get better. Some of the more common types of respiratory diseases include asthma, chronic obstructive lung disease, emphysema, lung cancer, complex lung infections, pulmonary hypertension and cystic fibrosis.

Heart disease

A cardiovascular disease specialist specializes in diseases of the heart and blood vessels and manages complex cardiac conditions such as heart attacks and life-threatening, abnormal heart rhythms. When it comes to treating heart disease, a patient may need to undergo a certain medical procedure, take one or more heart medications or make any necessary changes to their lifestyle that supports a healthy heart.

Hypertension

Hypertension means that a patient has high blood pressure in their arteries. These vessels play a very important role in one's overall health, as they carry blood from the heart to the rest of the body. When it comes to how internal medicine doctors treat hypertension, it depends on each individual patient. Two of the more common treatments for addressing hypertension in patients include taking prescribed medications and making any necessary lifestyle changes that support a healthy body.

内科学是临床医学的一个专科。它涵盖了心脏、肺、肾脏、肝脏、胰腺、甲状腺等器官的疾病。内科医生负责处理的疾病有糖尿病、高血压和高胆固醇等。

以下是一些最常见的内科疾病：

呼吸道疾病

普通内科医生以及呼吸内科专科医生经常帮助有呼吸系统问题的患者。他们为这些患者提供正确的诊断以及所需的治疗或管理服务，促使病情好转。常见的呼吸道疾病包括哮喘、慢性阻塞性肺病、肺气肿、肺癌、复杂肺部感染、肺动脉高压和囊性纤维化。

心脏疾病

心血管内科专家专门研究心脏和血管疾病，并处理复杂的心脏疾病，如心脏病急性发作和危及生命的心律失常。在治疗心脏疾病时，患者可能需要接受某种诊疗方案，服用一种或多种心脏药物，或对生活方式进行必要的改变，以保持心脏健康。

高血压

高血压是指患者动脉血压过高。血管在人体健康中扮演着非常重要的角色，因为它们将血液从心脏输送到身体的其他部位。内科医生如何治疗高血压取决于每位患者的具体情况。治疗高血压最常见的两种方法包括服用处方药和改变必要的生活方式以保持身体健康。

📋 Practical Activity

Work with your partner to create and perform a doctor-patient dialogue related to internal medicine diseases.

B. Practical Unit Project

Guidance for Production

Please work in groups and design a poster on "Preventing COVID-19". Then, make a presentation of your poster. For example, you can list guidelines on prevention of COVID-19 at supermarket or school; you can give health advice to people in the local area; or you can present regulations that people should observe during the pandemic.

Tips for designing a poster:

Step 1: Build your foundation.

- Who is my target viewer?
- Why would that person be interested in my poster?
- What kind of content would they most likely respond to?
- What are their needs, challenges, and pain points?
- What can my poster do for them?

Step 2: Draft an outline.

Create an outline to ensure any information you're presenting is clear, clean, and concise.

Step 3: Make artistic choices.

Make decisions on color scheme, images and text layout.

Step 4: Make sure your CTA (call to action) is easy to spot.

Make sure your CTA (call to action) is clear and visible to the reader.

Tips for making a presentation:

1. To deliver your presentation clearly, you need to be loud enough.

2. You need to use appropriate gestures and movements, make eye contact and use the right facial expressions.

3. When you get prepared for the presentation, rehearse delivering it to a classmate or a friend to see if there are any problems. Then revise the presentation before you deliver it in the class.

Part IV   Self-Assessment

Use the following self-assessment checklist to check what you have learned in this unit.

I understand the prevention of disease focusing on some specific measures.	☐
I can identify and use the words, phrases and sentence patterns related to the topic.	☐
I can make a poster by using the terminologies and medical information in this unit with my group members.	☐
I know how to understand the spirit of dedication.	☐

Unit 2
Healthy Living

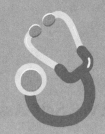

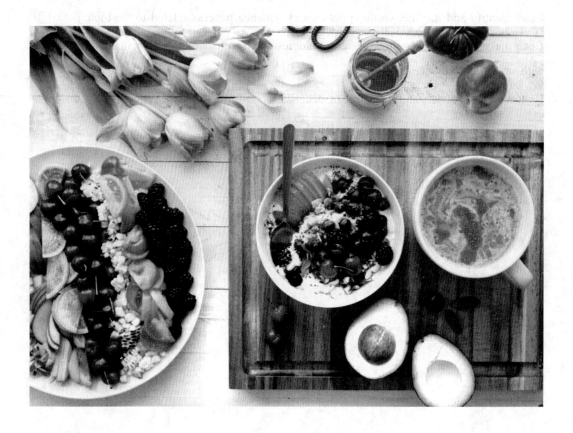

Healthy living is becoming a popular trend, and it is defined as a way of life that promotes physical, mental, and social well-being. A healthy lifestyle involves eating a balanced diet, engaging in regular physical activity, maintaining a good sleep pattern, and managing stress. Good nutrition is an indispensable part of leading a healthy lifestyle. Some foods, like avocados and olive oil, provide benefits to

Lead in

minds and bodies. If a person can successfully combine nutrition with health-related behaviors, this can help him or her to attain the right weight, diminish chances of suffering from diseases and enhance the overall health.

This unit is mainly to achieve the following objectives:

1) Understand different healthy behaviors that consist a healthy lifestyle;

2) Identify words, phrases and sentence patterns related to the topic;

3) Write an essay about healthy living lifestyle by using the terminologies and medical information in this unit;

4) Learn the importance of healthy living habits.

Part I　View the Medical World

Watch the video and choose the right answer.①

1. How many days did Randy Gardner stay awake?

　　A. 8.　　　　　　　　B. 9.　　　　　　　　C. 10.　　　　　　　　D. 11.

2. On which day did Randy Gardner lose the ability to distinguish objects by touch?

　　A. The 1st day.　　　B. The 2nd day.　　　C. The 3rd day.　　　D. The 4th day.

3. How much sleep do teenagers need?

　　A. 8 hours.　　　　　B. 9 hours.　　　　　C. 10 hours.　　　　　D. 11 hours.

4. What is NOT caused by sleep deprivation?

　　A. Diarrhea.　　　　B. Diabetes.　　　　C. Moody.　　　　　D. Poor memory.

5. What can clear out the brain's daily waste products?

　　A. Caffeine.　　　　　　　　　　　　　B. Adenosine.

　　C. Cerebrospinal fluid.　　　　　　　　D. Melatonin.

⊞ Words and Phrases

hallucinate /həˈluːsɪneɪt/ v. 产生幻觉

hormone /ˈhɔːməʊn/ n. 荷尔蒙

adenosine /əˈdenəsiːn/ n. 腺苷

melatonin /ˌmeləˈtəʊnɪn/ n. 褪黑素

inflammation /ˌɪnfləˈmeɪʃn/ n. 发炎

cerebrospinal /ˌserɪbrəʊˈspaɪnəl/ adj. 脑脊液的

lymphatic /lɪmˈfætɪk/ adj. 淋巴的

restorative /rɪˈstɔːrətɪv/ adj. 恢复健康的

---

① 视频详见网站:https://pan-yz. cldisk. com/external/m/file/1055138481566867456。

Part II   Read to Explore Medical Knowledge

Text A

Pre-reading Questions:

1. What is your understanding of healthy ageing?

2. What can we do to have a healthy ageing?

A Healthy Lifestyle Leads to Healthy Ageing

Text A

1. Throughout history, humanity has sought various methods and mystical elixirs to extend their lifespan. In the present era, the concepts of promoting a healthy ageing process are of worldwide significance and applicability, and are proved by scientific investigations. Based on WHO predictions, the global population of individuals aged 60 and beyond is projected to reach 2.1 billion by 2050, with 1.7 billion residing in low-income nations. The UN General Assembly has named 2021-2030 as the UN Decade of Healthy Ageing, so as to address the growing population of those aged 60 and above and to encourage longer and healthier lives. Given the global concern over population ageing, it is imperative to identify interventions that are both accessible and affordable in order to promote healthy ageing. Adopting a healthy lifestyle will likely be crucial.

2. The process of ageing is linked to the onset of numerous chronic ailments, including cardiovascular disorders and dementia. Animal studies have demonstrated that caloric restriction can decrease the occurrence of age-related chronic diseases and extend lifespan. William Kraus and his colleagues published a human study on medium-term caloric restriction in the September 2019 edition of *The Lancet Diabetes & Endocrinology*. The researchers divided the participants into two groups: a 25% caloric-restriction diet group

consisting of young and middle-aged individuals (aged 21-50 years) who were healthy and not obese, and an ad libitum control group. They then monitored these subjects for a period of 2 years. Caloric restriction resulted in an average decrease in calorie consumption of 11.9%. The participants in the caloric-restriction diet group experienced a consistent and significant decrease in all measured conventional cardiometabolic risk factors, such as LDL-cholesterol, total cholesterol to HDL-cholesterol ratio, and systolic and diastolic blood pressure, when compared to those in the control group. Moreover, there were no significant negative incidents reported, indicating that implementing a small reduction in calorie intake can be a secure and efficient measure to enhance cardiometabolic well-being. In the February 2022 edition of the journal *Science*, Olga Spadaro and her team conducted a detailed analysis of the data previously collected by Kraus and his colleagues. Their objective was to examine the impact of caloric restriction on immunometabolism. Thymopoiesis and induced pathways related to mitochondrial bioenergetics, anti-inflammatory responses, and lifespan were activated by 2 years of caloric restriction. These findings elucidate the mechanisms via which calorie restriction controls lifespan and have the potential to facilitate the development of targeted therapies for enhancing healthy ageing.

3. Drinking enough fluids may hasten the ageing process as well. In the January 2023 issue of *eBioMedicine*, Natalia Dmitrieva and colleagues found that middle-aged people (45-66 years old) who had high normal serum sodium levels (142 to <146 mmol/l) had a 39% increased risk of developing chronic diseases, such as heart failure, dementia, chronic lung diseases, and stroke. People in this range of serum sodium levels were up to 50% more likely to have an advanced biological age than their actual chronological age; this puts them at greater risk for developing chronic diseases and dying at a younger age. The results of this study provided support for the idea that increasing fluid consumption to maintain appropriate hydration could potentially slow down the ageing process, since serum sodium concentration has been used as a proxy for hydration status in healthy humans.

4. While caloric restriction is one way to maintain homoeostasis, increasing energy expenditure (via things like exercise) is another way to keep energy levels stable. It is necessary to develop a kind of physical exercise that is more suited to persons over the age of 60 in order to decrease mortality rates, since various forms of exercise call for different abilities. More than 270,000 participants, ranging in age from 59 to 82, were studied to determine the

associations between seven forms of physical activity and mortality rates from all causes, cardiovascular disease, and cancer. The activities included running, cycling, swimming, racquet sports, golf, walking for exercise, and other forms of aerobic exercise. The study was published in the August 2022 issue of the *JAMA Network Open*. There was a curvilinear dose-response relationship between mortality risk and each activity. Those who engaged in 7.5 to less than 15 metabolic equivalent of task (MET) hours a week of racquet sports and running had the lowest risk of all-cause mortality, compared to those who did not engage in any activity at all. The best risk reduction for cardiovascular mortality was found to be racquet sports, whereas the best risk reduction for cancer mortality was found to be running. Although there may be more hazards than benefits to being too active after 60, this study found that any activity from 7.5 to less than 15 MET hours per week reduced mortality chances, with racquet sports and jogging providing the greatest benefits.

5. The ageing process might be influenced by social factors. The biggest meta-analysis of the relationship between social connections and cognition at the individual participant level was published in the November 2022 issue of *The Lancet Healthy Longevity* by Suraj Samtani and colleagues. The study comprised thirteen longitudinal cohort studies conducted worldwide and involved over three hundred and eighty thousand individuals. Global cognitive, memory, and language decline was slowed by living with others rather than alone, and memory decline was slowed by engaging with community groups once a week and by interacting with family and friends once a week. These results highlight the significance of social connections for the psychological well-being of persons over the age of 60 and may inspire community and family members to provide more group activities for the elderly.

6. Various healthy practices should be integrated to form a healthy lifestyle. A prospective cohort of over 29,000 individuals older than 60 years old was studied to determine the effect of an ideal lifestyle on memory loss, one of the phenotypes in ageing. The results were published in the January 2023 issue of *BMJ* by Jianping Jia and colleagues. They looked at six aspects of a healthy lifestyle: what people eat, how often they exercise, how active they are socially and cognitively, whether they smoke or not, and whether they drink alcohol or not. The number of elements used to classify the participants into three groups: the advantageous (4-6 factors), the average (2-4 factors), and the unfavorable (0-1 factor). Memory deterioration was slower in the favorable and average groups compared to the

unfavorable group, regardless of apolipoprotein E ε4 status. The significance of maintaining a healthy lifestyle on neurocognitive health is emphasized in this study. Additional research is needed to see if it can influence other aspects of the ageing process.

7. There is still a lot we don't know about the ageing process, which is elusive. A longer life expectancy is just one of the goals of good ageing; other objectives include better mental and physical health as well as overall well-being for those over the age of 60. While living a healthy lifestyle isn't the only way to age well, it's one of the easier ones. The need to comprehend the processes of ageing and create treatments to avoid or postpone the commencement of age-related illnesses is of inereasingly great importance and urgency due to the increase in the population of individuals aged over 60.

New Words and Expressions

New Words and
Expressions

elixir /ɪˈlɪksər/ n. a substance believed to cure all illness 灵丹妙药

intervention /ˌɪntəˈvenʃn/ n. being involved in a situation in order to improve or help it 干预

accessible /əkˈsesəbl/ adj. that can be used, obtained, etc. 能使用的

onset /ˈɒnset/ n. the beginning of sth., especially sth. unpleasant 开端；肇始(尤指不快的事件)

cardiovascular /ˌkɑːdiəʊˈvæskjələ/ adj. relating to the heart and blood vessels 心血管的

dementia /dɪˈmenʃə/ n. a serious mental disorder caused by brain disease or injury, that affects the ability to think, remember and behave normally 痴呆

caloric /kəˈlɒrɪk/ adj. of or relating to calories in food 热量的

ad libitum /æd ˈlɪbɪtəm/ adv. without advance preparation 随意地

significant /sɪgˈnɪfɪkənt/ adj. large or important enough to have an effect or to be noticed 有重大意义的；显著的

cardiometabolic /ˈkɑːdiəʊˌmetəˈbɒlɪk/ adj. related to conditions and diseases that affect both the cardiovascular system (heart and blood vessels) and metabolic processes (such as glucose and lipid metabolism) 心血管代谢的

intake /ˈɪnteɪk/ *n.* the amount of food, drink, etc. that you take into your body 摄入量

immunometabolism /ɪmˈjunoʊməˈtæbəlɪzəm/ *n.* It describes the changes that occur in intracellular metabolic pathways in immune cells during activation. 免疫代谢

thymopoiesis /θaɪmɔpɔɪˈiːsis/ *n.* the process of development and maturation of T lymphocytes (also known as thymocytes) in the thymus gland 胸腺生成

induce /ɪnˈdjuːs/ *v.* to cause sth. 引起；导致

pathway /ˈpɑːθweɪ/ *n.* a way of achieving sth. 途径

mitochondrial bioenergetics /ˌmaɪtəʊˈkɒndriəl biːəʊnədˈʒetɪks/ 线粒体生物能量

anti-inflammatory /ˌænti ɪnˈflæmətri/ *adj.* (of a drug) used to reduce inflammation 抗炎的；消炎的

mechanism /ˈmekənɪzəm/ *n.* a system of parts in a living thing that together perform a particular function(生物体内的)机制；构造

serum sodium /ˈsɪərəm ˈsəʊdiəm/ *n.* the concentration of sodium ions in the blood serum, which is the clear, liquid component of blood that remains after red and white blood cells and platelets have been removed 血清钠

chronological /ˌkrɒnəˈlɒdʒɪkl/ *adj.* the number of years a person has lived as opposed to their level of physical, mental or emotional development 按时间计算的(年龄)(相对于身体、智力或情感等方面的发展而言)

concentration /ˌkɒnsnˈtreɪʃn/ *n.* the amount of a substance in a liquid or in another substance 浓度

proxy /ˈprɒksi/ *n.* something that you use to represent sth. else that you are trying to measure or calculate(测算用的)指标

hydration status /haɪˈdreɪʃn ˈsteɪtəs/ It refers to the amount of water and fluid balance in the body. It is a measure of how well-hydrated or dehydrated an individual is. 水合状态

homeostasis /ˌhəʊmiəˈsteɪsɪs/ *n.* the tendency towards a relatively stable equilibrium between interdependent elements, especially as maintained by physiological processes 体内平衡

expenditure /ɪkˈspendɪtʃə(r)/ *n.* the use of energy(精力的)消耗

curvilinear /ˌkɜːvɪˈlɪniə/ *adj.* consisting of a curved line or lines 曲线的

dose-response /dəʊs rɪˈspɒns/ *n.* a concept describes the effect of different doses or concentrations of a drug or substance on the magnitude of its response. This relationship illustrates how changes in the dose affect the biological effect produced by the drug. 剂量反应

meta-analysis /ˈmetə əˈnæləsɪs/ *n.* a method designed to increase the reliability of research by combining and analyzing the results of all known trials of the same product or experiments on the same subject 元分析

cognition /kɒɡˈnɪʃn/ *n.* mental process involved in knowing, learning, and understanding things 认知

longitudinal /ˌlɒŋɡɪˈtjuːdɪnl/ *adj.* concerning the development of sth. over a period of time 纵向的

cohort /ˈkəʊhɔːt/ *n.* a group who have sth. in common（有共同特点或举止类同的）一群人

prospective /prəˈspektɪv/ *adj.* expect to do sth. or become sth. 有望的；预期的；可能的

phenotype /ˈfiːnətaɪp/ *n.* the set of characteristics of a living thing, resulting from its combination of genes and the effect of its environment 表现型（基因和环境作用的结合而形成的一组生物特征）

favorable /ˈfeɪvərəbl/ *adj.* approving 有利的

apolipoprotein /ˌæpəˌlɪpəˈprəʊtɪn/ *n.* a protein that plays a crucial role in the transport and metabolism of lipids in the bloodstream 载脂蛋白

neurocognitive /ˌnjʊərəʊˈkɒɡnətɪv/ *adj.* related to both the nervous system and cognition 神经认知的

elusive /iˈluːsɪv/ *adj.* difficult to grasp by the mind or analyze 难以解释的；难以捉摸的

Notes

1. UN General Assembly：One of the six main agencies of the United Nations and the only one in which all member states of the United Nations participate. The United Nations General Assembly is held once a year and is primarily a deliberative body that can discuss and

propose suggestions on any issue within the scope of the United Nations Charter.

联合国大会是联合国六个主要机构之一，是唯一一个联合国所有成员国都参加的组织。联合国大会每年举行一次，它主要是一个审议机构，可以对《联合国宪章》规定范围内的任何问题进行讨论并提出建议。

2. chronic disease：The full name of chronic disease is a chronic non-infectious disease, which is a general name for a type of prolonged diseases that have hidden onset and long course, and is lacking of exact evidence of infectious biological etiology. The common chronic diseases include cancer, hypertension, coronary heart disease, diabetes, chronic respiratory disease, etc.

慢性病全称是慢性非传染性疾病，是对一类起病隐匿，病程长且病情迁延不愈，缺乏确切的传染性生物病因证据，病因复杂，且有些尚未完全被确认的疾病的概括性总称，如癌症、高血压、冠心病、糖尿病、慢性呼吸系统疾病等。

3. cardiometabolic risk factors：Metabolic risk factors are the main changeable risk factors leading to cardiovascular diseases, such as impaired glucose metabolism, dyslipidemia, hypertension, obesity, hyperuricemia, hyperhomocysteinemia. They may also cause metabolic disorders, systemic inflammation and oxidative stress, which ultimately lead to Atherosclerosis and cardiovascular disease.

心脏代谢危险因素是导致心血管疾病的主要可改变的危险因素，比如糖代谢受损、血脂异常、高血压、肥胖、高尿酸血症、高同型半胱氨酸血症，也是引起代谢失调、全身炎症、氧化应激的危险因素，这些因素最终导致了动脉粥样硬化和心血管病。

4. metabolic equivalent（MET）：Metabolic equivalent is the oxygen consumption required to maintain resting metabolism. It is a common indicator to express the relative energy metabolism level during various activities based on the energy consumption during quiet sitting, and can be used to evaluate the cardiopulmonary function.

代谢当量是维持静息代谢所需要的耗氧量。它是根据安静坐姿时的能量消耗来表示各种活动中相对能量代谢水平的常用指标，可用于评估心肺功能。

5. systolic and diastolic blood pressure：Systolic and diastolic blood pressure are the high and low pressures we refer to when measuring blood pressure in our daily lives. Systolic pressure refers to the pressure generated by the whole body's Great vessels when the heart contracts. The normal value is below 140mmHg and above 90mmHg; diastolic pressure refers

to the pressure of Great vessels in the whole body when the heart relaxes, which is below 90mmHg and above 60mmHg.

　　收缩压和舒张压就是我们日常测量血压时所说的高压与低压。收缩压指的是心脏收缩时全身大血管产生的压力，正常值在 140mmHg 以下，90mmHg 以上；舒张压指的是心脏舒张时全身大血管的压力大小，在 90mmHg 以下，60mmHg 以上。

▣ After Reading Activities

Reading Comprehension

✅ I. Answer the following questions.

1. What are the two major ways to promote healthy ageing mentioned in paragraph one?

2. What is the conclusion from the study about taking physical exercise for people older than 60?

3. How do social factors help to slow the ageing process?

4. What are the six healthy lifestyle factors mentioned in the text?

5. What are the goals of healthy ageing?

✅ II. Work in groups to complete the following chart according to the structure of the text.

Introduction and thesis statement: (para. 1)

　　As population ageing is becoming a global issue, finding ＿＿＿＿＿＿ and affordable interventions to promote healthy ageing will be ＿＿＿＿＿＿. Healthy lifestyle choices will probably be essential.

Accessible and affordable interventions and healthy lifestyle choices: (paras. 2-6)

1. Caloric restriction has been shown to reduce incidence of age-related ＿＿＿＿＿＿ ＿＿＿＿＿＿＿＿ rates and increase lifespan in animal studies. (para. 2)

2. Fluid intake could also contribute to the ageing process. A proper increase of fluid intake to maintain ＿＿＿＿＿＿＿＿ might slow the ageing process. (para. 3)

3. 7.5 to less than 15 MET hours per week of any activity is sufficient to reduce ＿＿＿＿＿＿, with racquet sports and running being the most beneficial. (para. 4)

4. Living with other people, _____ with family and friends and community group engagement predicted slower global cognitive, memory and language decline than living alone. (para. 5)

5. A healthy lifestyle is an integration of different healthy behaviors, which is important for _____ health. (para. 6)

Conclusion: (para. 7)

A healthy lifestyle can be an easy way to promote healthy ageing. Understanding the _____ of ageing and developing interventions to prevent or delay the onset of age associated diseases are becoming increasingly important and urgent.

Words and Phrases

✅ I. Translate the following medical terms into Chinese or English.

1. serum sodium level   _____

2. neurocognitive health   _____

3. anti-inflammatory response   _____

4. metabolic equivalent   _____

5. 水合状态   _____

6. 剂量反应   _____

7. 收缩压和舒张压   _____

8. 心脏代谢危险因素   _____

✅ II. Fill in the blanks with the words or phrases given below. Change the form if necessary.

expenditure	induce	concentration	prospective	favorable

1. The chemist carefully measured the _____ of salt in the water to ensure the experiment's accuracy.

2. _____ policies are in effect to encourage employee's professional development.

3. _____ on health in most of these countries has gone down, and the same is true for education.

4. The harsh critics' comments _____ a strong response from the artist, leading to a series of defensive interviews.

5. As medical students, it is important to stay motivated throughout your studies. A clear career _____ can help you maintain focus and dedication to your long-term goals.

Sentence Translation

Translate the following sentences into Chinese or English.

1. The participants in the caloric-restriction diet group experienced a consistent and significant decrease in all measured conventional cardiometabolic risk factors, such as LDL-cholesterol, total cholesterol to HDL-cholesterol ratio, and systolic and diastolic blood pressure, when compared to those in the control group.

_____

_____

2. Middle-aged people (45-66 years old) who had normal serum sodium levels that were high (142 to <146 mmol/l) were 39% more likely to develop chronic diseases, such as heart failure, dementia, chronic lung diseases, and stroke.

_____

_____

3. While caloric restriction is one way to maintain homoeostasis, increasing energy expenditure (via things like exercise) is another way to keep energy levels stable.

_____

_____

4. 与他人而非独自生活可减缓整体认知、记忆和语言能力的下降速度，每周参加一次社区小组活动以及每周与家人和朋友交流一次可减缓记忆力的下降速度。

_____

_____

5. 由于 60 岁以上人口的增加，了解衰老过程和创造治疗方法以避免或推迟老年相关疾病的发生变得越来越重要和迫切。

_____

_____

Text B

Pre-reading Questions:

1. What is nutrition intervention?

2. What is the impact of nutrition intervention?

3. How can physicians and governments promote public health through nutrition intervention?

Eat Well to Live Well

Text B

1. For lasting health, the golden rule—"eat healthy to live healthy"—can be a fundamental mantra. From prenatal development all the way into adulthood, this Special Issue seeks to discuss the obstacles faced by preventative efforts that rely on nutritional treatments and behavioral changes, from fetus to adulthood. Even maternal nutrition, which is known to increase the likelihood of troubles during pregnancy, appears to be a role in the development of intergenerational health issues in offspring.

2. Adequate nutrition is of the utmost importance throughout the years of infancy and childhood, a time marked by both fast physical and mental development and the establishment of foundational skills for the rest of a person's life. Here, the length of time a baby spends nursing and receiving supplemental food plays a significant influence in shaping their taste preferences and habits, which might lead to a decreased likelihood of developing long-term health problems like obesity.

3. The epigenetic effects and low protein content of breast milk make it the most essential factor in reducing juvenile obesity during the first few months of life.

4. Providing moms with appropriate information throughout pregnancy and after birth is crucial in helping them initiate and continue breastfeeding. When a mother starts nursing, she may be more vulnerable to the adverse effects of stressful circumstances. Nursing success may be affected by stress caused by hospitalization, according to a new study by Foligno et al., especially in intensive care units and during extended hospital stays.

5. A baby's diet resembles that of other members of the family after the first year. Choosing

foods that are safe and high-quality for young children is still an important consideration. The food consumption habits of families have unfortunately become habitual, which can have negative impacts on health. Non-communicable chronic illnesses have been on the rise, particularly in developing nations, due to the widespread preference for calorie-rich diets with low nutritional value over nutritious foods high in micronutrients.

6. D'Auria et al. evaluate data on how supplemental eating affects the development of chronic non-communicable illnesses, and they offer advice on how to eat supplementally healthily.

7. A population-based survey by Baldassarre et al. shows that, during complementary feeding, people are increasingly adopting diets that they view as healthier, even when they are not under the supervision of specialist physicians. Severe dietary deficiencies might have detrimental long-term implications, which must be taken into account in such circumstances.

8. Alcohol intake during adolescence is common among harmful habits that people acquire and continue throughout their lives. "Binge drinking," defined as consuming an excessive amount of alcohol in a short period of time, is one form of excessive drinking that contributes significantly to global health concerns. Kim et al. found that 52% of male and female Korean college students binge drink, which can lead to a variety of negative outcomes including health problems (both acute and chronic), accidents, and antisocial conduct. Among other things, the scientists discovered a correlation between exercise and alcohol intake, and they used this and other findings to propose measures to curb alcohol abuse.

9. Lowering expenses and improving health and quality of life may be achieved via the intake of health foods. Adults are more likely to acquire healthy eating habits if their companies provide them with food (staff canteens) throughout the workday that is balanced and prepared in accordance with current norms.

10. A recent research by Czarniecka-Skubina et al. underscores the relevance of workplace nutrition as a possible essential intervention to lower the prevalence of chronic illnesses in adult populations and enhance public health via direct and indirect measures. Among the factors that contribute to emotional weariness, work satisfaction, and organizational behavior, the authors emphasized the significance of taking breaks. The authors compared five Warsaw staff canteens that were comparable in terms of size, seating capacity, and

daily meal serving volume. Their findings have real-world consequences for those in charge of staff cafeterias: consumers keep tabs on "healthy" diet trends and assume that cafeterias will start serving healthier options, highlighting the need to expand menu diversity to include more vegetarian and vegan options as well as healthful dishes.

11. In order to promote public health habits, it is necessary to enhance health food marketing techniques and interventions for groups at high risk.

12. In this regard, health food marketing tactics might borrow from the findings of a fascinating study conducted by Lee et al. The individuals the writers set out to reach were those who had invested in health food items with the intention of enhancing their digestive systems. The authors proved that repurchase intention was positively affected by perceptions of vulnerability, severity, action advantages, and behavioral control.

13. The study by Sato et al. shows that the fast-growing market for dietary supplements—which include pills, powders, granules, or liquids with functional physiological ingredients different from those in regular food—is of great interest for the development of health food marketing strategies.

14. In ageing society, people are hoping that dietary supplements, which are a kind of self-medication, will help promote health and avoid disease. Within the regulatory framework, dietary supplements fall somewhere in the middle, between food and medication. Standardized procedures for the production of dietary supplements are promoted and carried out in accordance with Good Manufacturing Practice (GMP). Research out of Japan by Sato et al. shows that pharmaceutical competence and experience making a variety of dietary supplement items affect the quality of such supplements.

15. Additional research on dietary and natural approaches to managing chronic non-communicable diseases is necessary. Nutraceuticals and functional foods are natural alternatives to pharmaceuticals that can enhance health and well-being while decreasing health care expenditures. According to the review by Idrus et al., honey was found to have a preventive impact against cardiovascular disease, which is a big public health burden globally.

16. Alginate-based formulations from brown algae were successfully used as a first therapy option for babies with chronic gastrointestinal discomfort due to gastroesophageal reflux (GER) in a study by Baldassarre et al., which suggests that additional treatments and

testing may not be necessary.

17. The potential roles of lifestyle and nutritional treatments in preventing human illness throughout all life stages have been demonstrated. In this special issue, we look at several behaviors and trends that might aid doctors in their work and governments in their efforts to promote healthy lifestyles via prevention.

New Words and Expressions

New Words and
Expressions

mantra /ˈmæntrə/ *n.* literally a sacred utterance in Vedism 颂歌

nutritional /njuˈtrɪʃənl/ *adj.* of or relating to or providing nutrition 营养成分的

fetus /fiːtəs/ *n.* an unborn or unhatched vertebrate in the later stages of development showing the main recognizable features of the mature animal 胎儿

maternal /məˈtɜːnl/ *adj.* relating to or derived from one's mother 母亲的

offspring /ˈɒfsprɪŋ/ *n.* a child of a particular person or couple 后代

infancy /ˈɪnfənsi/ *n.* the time when a child is a baby or very young 婴儿期

obesity /əʊˈbiːsɪti/ *n.* more than average fatness 肥胖

epigenetic /ˌepɪdʒɪˈnetɪk/ *adj.* of or relating to epigenesis 表观遗传学的；后生的

protein /ˈprəʊtiːn/ *n.* a substance found in food and drink such as meat, eggs, and milk 蛋白质

hospitalization /ˌhɒspɪtəlaɪˈzeɪʃ(ə)n/ *n.* placing in medical care in a hospital 住院治疗

resemble /rɪˈzembl/ *v.* to look like or be similar to another person or thing 像；相似

consumption /kənˈsʌmpʃn/ *n.* the act of using energy, food or materials 消耗

micronutrient /ˌmaɪkrəʊˈnjuːtrɪənt/ *n.* a substance needed only in small amounts for normal body function 微量营养素

deficiency /dɪˈfɪʃnsi/ *n.* lack of an adequate quantity or number 不足；缺乏

detrimental /ˌdetrɪˈmentl/ *adj.* causing harm or injury 有害的

implication /ˌɪmplɪˈkeɪʃn/ *n.* a possible effect or result of an action or a decision 可能的影响

adolescence /ˌædəˈlesns/ *n.* in the state that someone is in between puberty and adulthood 青春期

excessive /ɪkˈsesɪv/ *adj.* beyond normal limits 过度的

acute /əˈkjuːt/ *adj.* an acute illness is one that has quickly become severe and dangerous 急性的

vegetarian /vedʒəˈteəriən/ *n.* a person who does not eat meat or fish 素食主义者

severity /sɪˈverəti/ *n.* sth. hard to endure 严重

supplement /ˈsʌplɪmənt/ *n.* a thing that is added to sth. else to improve or complete it 补充物；增补物

granule /ˈɡrænjuːl/ *n.* a small, hard piece of sth. ; a small grain 颗粒

ingredient /ɪnˈɡriːdiənt/ *n.* one of the things from which sth. is made, especially one of the foods that are used together to make a particular dish 成分

self-medication /self ˌmedɪˈkeɪʃn/ *n.* the use of medicine without medical supervision to treat one's own ailments 自我治疗

pharmaceutical /fɑːməˈsuːtɪkl/ *adj.* connected with making and selling drugs and medicines 制药的

alternative /ɔːlˈtɜːnətɪv/ *n.* a thing that you can choose to do or have out of two or more possibilities 可供选择的事物

alginate /ˈældʒɪˌneɪt/ *n.* a salt or ester of alginic acid 海藻盐酸

algae /ˈældʒiː/ *n.* very simple plants with no real leaves, stems or roots that grow in or near water, including seaweed 海藻

gastrointestinal /ɡæstrəʊɪnˈtestɪnl/ *adj.* of or related to the stomach and intestines 胃肠的

gastroesophageal /ˈɡæstrəʊɪsɔfəˈdʒiːəl/ *adj.* of or relating to or involving the stomach and esophagus 胃食管的

reflux /ˈriːflʌks/ *n.* an abnormal backward flow of body fluids 反流

🗏 Notes

1. mantra：The Sanskrit Mantra is translated as "mandala", also known as "mantra" or "maxim". They are the voices that ancient yoga masters perceived in deep meditation to have a positive impact on the body and mind of humans.

梵文 Mantra 被译为"曼陀罗"，也被译为"咒语"或"箴言"。它们是古代瑜伽大师们在

深度冥想中感知到的对人的身体和心灵具有积极影响的声音。

2. epigenetic effect：Epigenetic effect is a botanical term published in 2019. Under the premise of not changing the DNA sequence, some mechanisms such as DNA methylation and histone acetylation can cause heritable gene expression or cell phenotype changes.

表观遗传学效应是 2019 年公布的植物学名词。在不改变 DNA 序列的前提下,通过某些机制如 DNA 甲基化、组蛋白乙酰化等引起可遗传的基因表达或细胞表型的变化。

3. binge drinking：Binge drinking is usually used to describe an unhealthy drinking behavior, especially when drinking heavily in a short period of time. It is usually associated with alcoholism and alcohol addictive behavior.

通常用来描述一种不健康的饮酒行为,尤其是在较短的时间内大量饮酒。它通常与酗酒和酒精成瘾行为相关联。

4. dietary supplements：Dietary supplements are used in biochemical research and as a dietary supplement. They contain one or more dietary ingredients, including vitamins, minerals, herbs, *or plants with practical use due* to their aroma, taste, or health characteristics.

膳食补充剂被用于生物化学研究,也是一种饮食添加剂。含有一种或多种膳食成分,包括维生素、矿物质、草药或者由于其香气、味道或者健康特性而具有使用价值的植物。

5. GMP：Good Manufacturing Practice was first promulgated by the United States Congress in 1963 to regulate drug production. This is also the world's first GMP. Due to the significant effectiveness of GMP in regulating drug production, improving drug quality, and ensuring drug safety, the Food and Drug Administration of the United States (FDA) issued the Food GMP in 1980 to regulate food production.

良好生产规范最早是美国国会为了规范药品生产而于 1963 年颁布的。这也是世界上第一部良好生产规范。由于良好生产规范在规范药品的生产,提高药品的质量,保证药品的安全方面效果非常明显,美国食品药品监督管理局(FDA)于 1980 年颁布了食品良好生产规范,用以规范食品的生产。

6. GER：gastroesophageal reflux refers to the reflux of gastric contents into the esophagus, which can be acidic, alkaline, or neutral.

胃食管反流指胃内食物反流至食管,反流物可以是酸性、碱性或中性的。

🗐 After Reading Activities

Reading Comprehension

Decide whether the following statements are true (T) or false (F) according to the text.

_____ 1. "Eat healthy to live healthy" is a fundamental mantra for short-term wellbeing.

_____ 2. The duration of breastfeeding exerts the sole role in establishing flavor preferences and behaviors.

_____ 3. Binge drinking is a leading cause of health problems worldwide.

_____ 4. Nutrition is a key intervention to reduce the incidence of chronic diseases in adult populations.

_____ 5. A food supplement is expected to contribute to promoting health and preventing disease of the elderly.

Words and Phrases

Match each English phrase in Column A with its Chinese version in Column B.

Column A	Column B
1. intensive care	A. 慢性疾病
2. adverse effects	B. 酒精滥用
3. calorie-rich	C. 均衡的饮食
4. chronic disease	D. 不良影响
5. binge drinking	E. 保健食品
6. alcohol abuse	F. 高热量的
7. a balanced diet	G. 酗酒
8. dietary supplements	H. 重症监护

Translation

　　健康饮食不必过于复杂。似乎并不只有你一人被互相矛盾的营养和饮食建议弄得晕头转向。你会发现只要有专家介绍某种食物对身体的好处，就会出现另一种相反的意见。尽管一些特定的食物或营养素已证明对情绪有好处，但整体饮食模式才是最重要的。健康饮食的基石是尽可能用天然食品替代加工食品。吃纯天然或准天然食品对你的思维、外表和情绪都能产生巨大的影响。

_____

_____

_____

_____

Critical Thinking

　　A healthy, balanced diet is usually less appealing and preferred to unhealthy food that has poor nutritional value. Please work in groups to have a discussion on adding more vegetables and fruits to your diet and how to make a healthy diet tasty and appealing.

Part III Apply Medical English

✅ A. Situational Dialogues in Different Clinical Departments

Dialogue

Pediatrics（儿科）

Diarrhea（腹泻）

Doctor：Sit down, please. What seems to be the problem with your child?

Patient：I am afraid he has loose bowels.

Doctor：How old is he?

Patient：Two years old.

Doctor：When did his diarrhea start?

Patient：He has had it for two days.

Doctor：Do you remember how many times did he go to the toilet?

Patient：I can't remember exactly. It must have been over six times.

Doctor：What kind of stool did you notice, watery or mucous?

Patient：They are quite loose with milk curd and undigested food in them.

Doctor：How about his urine? How many times a day?

Patient：About 6 to 7 times a day.

Doctor：Is he losing weight?

Patient：No. Everything else seems to be all right.

Doctor：Does he have any other problems?

Patient：He runs a low temperature of about 37.8℃ and he has a poor appetite.

Doctor：Can you tell me his dietary history?

Patient：Yes, doctor. His diet is as usual, for instance, congee, milk, egg, rice, etc..

Doctor：Is he allergic to milk?

Patient：No, he isn't.

Doctor：Is he a breastfed infant?

Patient：Yes. I gave him the breast till he was one year old.

Doctor：What about his parturition, natural or medicated?

Patient：The puerperal process is natural.

Doctor：Did he suffer from other diseases before?

Patient：He is healthy always, and scarcely feel sick.

Doctor：I think the diarrhea probably was caused by virus infection. Please don't stop food and milk, encourage him to take food, and feed him more times than usual. I will prescribe some medicine and ORS (oral rehydration salt) for him to prevent dehydration.

Patient：Is the disease serious, doctor?

Doctor：No, not so serious. With proper treatment, he'll get better gradually.

Patient：That's a relief. Thank you very much, doctor.

Words and Phrases

have loose bowels /hæv luːs ˈbaʊəlz/ 拉肚子

diarrhea /ˌdaɪəˈriːə/ *n.* 腹泻

mucous /ˈmjuːkəs/ *adj.* 黏液的

milk curd /mɪlk kɜːd/ 凝乳

dietary /ˈdaɪətəri/ *adj.* 饮食的

breastfeed infant /ˈbrestfiːd ˈɪnfənt/ 母乳喂养的婴儿

parturition /ˌpɑːtjuˈrɪʃn/ *n.* 分娩

puerperal /pjʊˈɜːpərəl/ *adj.* 分娩的

medicated /ˈmedɪkeɪtɪd/ *adj.* 用药治疗的

ORS (oral rehydration salt) /ˈɔːrəli ˌriːhaɪˈdreɪʃn sɔːlt/ 补液盐

dehydration /ˌdiːhaɪˈdreɪʃən/ *n.* 脱水

Notes

✅ 1. Here are some common pediatric diseases：

Respiratory Infections

Respiratory infections, including the common cold, flu, bronchitis, and pneumonia, are frequent occurrences in children, particularly in infants and toddlers.

Gastrointestinal Infections

Gastrointestinal infections such as gastroenteritis (stomach flu) and rotavirus are common in children, leading to symptoms like diarrhea, vomiting, and abdominal pain.

Ear Infections

Otitis media, or middle ear infections, are common in young children, often occurring after a cold or respiratory infection. Symptoms include ear pain, fever, and fussiness.

Asthma

Asthma is a chronic respiratory condition characterized by inflammation and narrowing of the airways, leading to wheezing, coughing, and difficulty breathing. It often begins in childhood and can be triggered by various factors, including allergens and respiratory infections.

Allergies

Allergic conditions such as allergic rhinitis (hay fever), eczema, and food allergies are common in children and can cause symptoms like sneezing, itching, rash, and difficulty breathing.

Skin Infections

Skin infections like impetigo, ringworm, and yeast infections are common in children, especially those who spend time in close contact settings like schools and daycare centers.

Childhood Obesity

Childhood obesity is a growing concern worldwide and can lead to various health problems, including type 2 diabetes, high blood pressure, and heart disease.

Attention-Deficit/Hyperactivity Disorder (ADHD)

ADHD is a common neurodevelopmental disorder in children, characterized by symptoms such as hyperactivity, impulsivity, and difficulty paying attention.

Autism Spectrum Disorder (ASD)

ASD is a developmental disorder that affects communication, social interaction, and behavior. It typically appears in early childhood and varies widely in severity.

Childhood Cancer

While relatively rare compared to other conditions, childhood cancer, including leukemia, lymphoma, and brain tumors, can occur and require specialized treatment.

以下是一些常见的儿科疾病：

呼吸道感染

呼吸道感染包括普通感冒、流感、支气管炎和肺炎，在儿童中经常发生，尤其是在婴幼儿期。

消化道感染

消化道感染如胃肠炎（胃部流感）和轮状病毒感染在儿童中常见，导致腹泻、呕吐和腹痛等症状。

耳道感染

中耳炎或称中耳感染，常见于幼儿，往往发生在感冒或呼吸道感染后。症状包括耳痛、发热和烦躁不安。

哮喘

哮喘是一种慢性呼吸道疾病，特征是气道炎症和狭窄，导致喘鸣、咳嗽和呼吸困难。它往往始于童年，并且可以被各种因素触发，包括过敏原和呼吸道感染。

过敏

过敏性疾病如过敏性鼻炎（花粉热）、湿疹和食物过敏在儿童中很常见，可导致打喷嚏、瘙痒、皮疹和呼吸困难等症状。

皮肤感染

皮肤感染如湿疹、癣和酵母感染等皮肤感染在儿童中常见，尤其是那些在学校和托儿所等密集接触环境中的儿童。

儿童肥胖

儿童肥胖是全球日益关注的问题，可能导致各种健康问题，包括 2 型糖尿病、高血压和心脏病。

注意力缺陷/多动障碍（ADHD）

ADHD 是一种常见的神经发育障碍，特征是多动、冲动和注意力不集中等症状。

自闭症谱系障碍（ASD）

ASD 是一种影响沟通、社交互动和行为的发育障碍。它通常在幼儿期出现，并且在严重程度上有很大的差异。

儿童癌症

虽然与其他疾病相比相对较少见，但儿童癌症，包括白血病、淋巴瘤和脑瘤，仍可能会发生，并且需要专门的治疗。

✅ 2. Pediatricians follow certain rules and strategies to establish rapport, build trust, and ensure clear communication with their young patients. Here are some rules for pediatricians to communicate with children:

- Use Age-Appropriate Language: Pediatricians use language that is simple, clear, and age-appropriate for the child's developmental level. They avoid medical jargon and explain concepts in a way that children can understand.

- Establish Rapport and Trust: Pediatricians take time to establish rapport and build trust with their young patients. They greet children warmly, engage them in conversation, and create a friendly and welcoming environment in the exam room.

- Encourage Participation: Pediatricians encourage children to participate in their health care by asking questions, expressing their concerns, and sharing their experiences. They listen actively to children's responses and validate their feelings and perspectives.

- Provide Reassurance and Comfort: Pediatricians provide reassurance and comfort to children who may be anxious or scared about medical visits or procedures. They offer praise and encouragement for cooperation and bravery and address any fears or misconceptions the child may have.

- Use Play and Distraction Techniques: Pediatricians use play and distraction techniques to help children feel more comfortable and relaxed during medical examinations and procedures. This may include using toys, books, or interactive games to engage the child and minimize anxiety.

- Respect Privacy and Boundaries: Pediatricians respect children's privacy and boundaries during medical examinations and discussions. They ensure that the child feels safe and comfortable and provide opportunities for the child to ask questions or raise concerns privately if needed.

- Involve Parents or Caregivers: Pediatricians involve parents or caregivers in the communication process, especially for younger children or those with limited verbal skills. They provide information and instructions to parents in a clear and understandable manner and encourage them to support their child's participation in health care decisions.

- Use Visual Aids: Pediatricians may use visual aids such as diagrams, pictures, or models to explain medical concepts or procedures to children. Visual aids can help reinforce verbal explanations and enhance understanding.

- Follow the Child's Lead: Pediatricians follow the child's lead during interactions, allowing them to express themselves at their own pace and comfort level. They adapt their communication style and approach based on the child's individual personality and preferences.
- Offer Positive Reinforcement: Pediatricians offer positive reinforcement and praise to children for their cooperation, participation, and efforts to take care of their health. Positive reinforcement helps build confidence and motivation for continued engagement in health care.

　　儿科医生遵循一定的规则和策略来与小患者建立融洽和信任的关系,并确保和小患者实现清晰的沟通。以下是儿科医生与儿童沟通的规则:

- 用适龄语言:儿科医生使用简单、清晰并适合儿童发育水平的语言。他们避免使用医学术语,并以儿童能够理解的方式解释概念。
- 建立融洽关系和信任关系:儿科医生花时间与小患者建立融洽和信任关系。他们热情地问候孩子,与他们交谈,并在检查室内营造一个友好和温馨的环境。
- 鼓励参与:儿科医生鼓励儿童通过提问、表达他们的担忧和分享他们的经历来参与他们的医疗护理。他们积极倾听孩子的回应,认可他们的感受和观点。
- 提供安慰和舒适的感觉:儿科医生为可能对问诊或治疗过程感到焦虑或害怕的儿童提供安慰和舒适的感觉。他们对孩子的合作和勇敢给予表扬和鼓励,并解决孩子可能存在的任何恐惧或误解。
- 使用游戏和分散注意力的技巧:儿科医生使用游戏和分散注意力的技巧,帮助孩子在医疗检查和治疗期间感到更加舒适和放松。这可能包括使用玩具、书籍或互动游戏来吸引孩子,减少焦虑。
- 尊重隐私和界限:儿科医生在医疗检查和讨论期间尊重孩子的隐私和界限。他们确保孩子感到安全和舒适,并在需要时提供机会让孩子私下提问或表达担忧。
- 让父母或看护人参与:儿科医生让父母或看护人参与沟通过程,特别是对于年龄较小或语言表达能力有限的儿童。他们以清晰易懂的方式向父母提供信息和指导,并鼓励他们支持孩子参与医疗决策。
- 使用视觉辅助工具:儿科医生可能使用图表、图片或模型等视觉辅助工具向孩子解释医疗概念或过程。视觉辅助工具可以帮助强化口头解释并增强理解。
- 跟随孩子的引导:儿科医生在互动过程中跟随孩子的引导,让孩子们以自己的节奏和舒适度来表达自己。医生根据孩子的个性和偏好调整他们的沟通风格和方法。

- 提供积极的强化鼓励：儿科医生对孩子的合作、参与以及他们对自己健康的努力给予积极的强化和表扬。积极的强化鼓励有助于孩子建立信心，并提供继续参与医疗的动力。

📇 Practical Activity

Work with your partner to create and perform a doctor-patient dialogue related to pediatric diseases.

✅ B. Practical Unit Project

Suppose you are writing a letter to Su Shi, giving your suggestions about healthier diet and drinking less. Also, you can give him more suggestions on how to live a healthy lifestyle. Try to use the expressions you've learned from this unit.

Guidance for Production

Steps for writing a letter of advice: write your letter step-by-step

Step 1: Explain that you are responding to a request for advice about a problem or situation.

Sample Sentences for Step 1

- *I am honored that you would ask me for advice on such an issue.*
- *I have been thinking about the schooling dilemma that we talked about.*
- *After talking with some of the former employees of Doe Realty, I think I can answer your question.*
- *Thank you for your letter asking for my opinion on how to proceed with your proposal.*
- *I've been thinking a lot about what you asked me last night.*
- *I've been considering the unhappy personal situation that you explained to me, and its impact on your work.*
- *After thinking about your problem for the past two days, I think you might want to consider a different approach.*

Step 2: Give your advice or suggestions.

Sample Sentences for Step 2

- *I really think that you should stay in school, even though you may have to take out a loan.*
- *It seems to me that you have done all you can short of seeing a professional counselor. I*

think that talking with such a counselor may be worthwhile. I have a recommendation, if you want to follow that course of action.

- *I believe your resume would be more effective if you would list your work experience with single one-line statements beginning with active verbs. For example, "Ensured quality control of product."*

- *Because your decision will have long-range consequences, I suggest that you speak to your minister before taking such a serious step.*

- *At your age you should begin to save as much as possible for retirement.*

- *Since Dr. Doe has spent most of his life in general practice, he may not be experienced with your special situation. I would recommend that you see a specialist for a second opinion.*

Step 3: Explain the reasons why you feel the way you do.

Sample Sentences for Step 3

- *The extra expense of finishing school now will be made up many times over in the next few years. Long-term studies show that the income of college graduates is significantly higher than that of non-graduates.*

- *Sometimes we are too close to a problem to see the solution. A third party can be a valuable aid to persons who genuinely want to solve a difficult problem.*

- *The use of strong verbs in this way conveys a crisp, effective message that gives the reader the feeling that the writer is competent.*

- *I think you need to consider the consequences for your children, as well as for your own emotional stability.*

- *A small percentage of your income invested each month will provide a significant return over a period of thirty years. You will probably need such savings to complement your regular retirement and possible social security payments.*

- *You shouldn't worry about Dr. Doe's reaction. You should be in charge of your own health, and he must understand that you need more information.*

Step 4: Add a comment that releases the reader from feeling an obligation to follow your advice.

Sample Sentences for Step 4

- *Of course, this is my personal opinion. Others may disagree.*

- *What I have written comes from my own experience. There may be factors that make your case different.*

- *I like this approach but you may want to look at others as well.*
- *Of course, this decision must be your own. I have only given you my opinion.*
- *There may be other ways of accomplishing your long-range financial goals. This one has worked for me, but it may not be the one for you.*
- *Of course, you are closer to the situation than I am, so there may be other factors that I have not taken into consideration.*

Step 5. Close with a note of encouragement and confidence.

Sample Sentences for Step 5

- *I think you are on the right track and will make the right choice.*
- *You have a good sense of right and wrong, so I am confident that you will make the right choice.*
- *You have been so meticulous in preparing this document that I am confident that the end result will be good.*
- *You are wise to get input from others before making a decision.*
- *After you have had a chance to talk with him, I feel that you will be able to make a wise decision.*
- *You are smart to begin planning this way in your early years. With such foresight, you will undoubtedly succeed.*
- *I wish you success in whatever decision you make. You certainly deserve it.*

Tips for living a healthy lifestyle:

1. Healthy Eating Habits:

- Focus on whole, unprocessed foods such as fruits, vegetables, whole grains, lean proteins, and healthy fats.
- Incorporate a variety of colors into your meals to ensure you're getting a wide range of nutrients.
- Limit added sugars, salt, and saturated fats in your diet by choosing foods with minimal processing and reading nutrition labels carefully.
- Practice portion control to avoid overeating and maintain a healthy weight.
- Stay hydrated by drinking plenty of water throughout the day.

2. Reduce Alcohol Consumption:

- Set limits on how much alcohol you consume and stick to them.

- Choose lower-alcohol options such as light beer or wine spritzers, and alternate alcoholic drinks with water or non-alcoholic beverages.
- Be mindful of the size of your drinks and avoid oversized servings.
- Consider the impact of alcohol on your overall health and well-being, and prioritize moderation.

3. Regular Physical Activity:

- Aim for at least 150 minutes of moderate-intensity aerobic activity or 75 minutes of vigorous-intensity activity per week, as recommended by health guidelines.
- Find activities you enjoy, such as walking, swimming, cycling, dancing, or playing sports, and incorporate them into your routine.
- Include strength training exercises at least two days per week to build muscle mass and improve overall fitness.
- Stay active throughout the day by incorporating movement into your daily activities, such as taking the stairs instead of the elevator or going for short walks during breaks.

4. Prioritize Sleep:

- Aim for 7-9 hours of quality sleep each night to support overall health and well-being.
- Establish a regular sleep schedule by going to bed and waking up at the same time every day, even on weekends.
- Create a relaxing bedtime routine to signal to your body that it's time to wind down, such as reading a book, taking a warm bath, or practicing relaxation techniques like deep breathing or meditation.
- Create a comfortable sleep environment by keeping your bedroom dark, quiet, and cool.

5. Stress Management:

- Practice stress-reducing techniques such as mindfulness meditation, yoga, deep breathing exercises, or progressive muscle relaxation.
- Identify sources of stress in your life and develop healthy coping strategies to manage them, such as problem-solving, seeking support from friends or family, or engaging in enjoyable activities.
- Prioritize self-care activities that promote relaxation and well-being, such as spending time in nature, engaging in hobbies, or spending quality time with loved ones.

Part IV   Self-Assessment

Use the following self-assessment checklist to check what you have learned in this unit.

I understand different healthy behaviors that consist a healthy lifestyle.	☐
I can identify and use the words, phrases and sentence patterns related to the topic.	☐
I can write an essay about healthy living lifestyle by using the terminologies and medical information in this unit.	☐
I understand the importance of healthy living habits.	☐

Unit 3
Health Care System

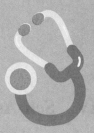

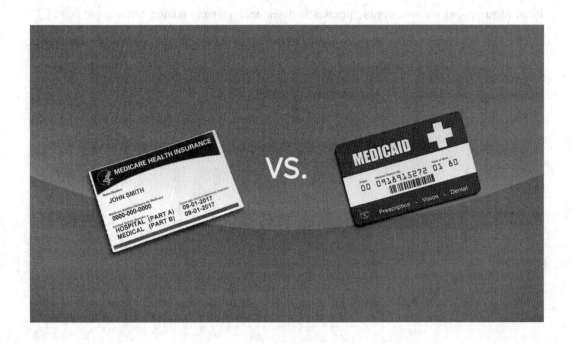

The primary function of health systems is to provide high-quality and universal health services. At the same time, through their spending and investments, health systems play an important role in the status and stability of national and regional economies. To date, this economic contribution has not been captured. Health systems play an increasingly important role in driving inclusive and sustainable development through responsible practices in the areas of employment and the purchasing of goods and services. This social benefit of health systems is not well documented or currently considered in many mainstream policies and practices.

Lead in

Health and well-being contribute to economic and social progress, and in turn, economic security and social cohesion are two key determinants of health.

This unit is mainly to achieve the following objectives:

1) Understand the basic concept and structure of health care system in the U.S.;

2) Identify words, phrases and sentence patterns related to the topic;

3) Understand and write an essay about how to confront challenges of health care system in the U.S.;

4) Compare the differences of health care system between China and the U.S.

Part I　View the Medical World

Watch a video about the history of the U.S. health care system and fill in the blanks.①

1. The Membership of the American Medical Association goes from about _____ physicians in 1900 to _____ in 1910.

　　A. 8,000；70,000　　B. 1,940；8,000　　C. 1,930；70,000　　D. 7,000；8,000

2. _____ changes the countries priorities to a greater emphasis on unemployment and old-age benefits.

　　A. The Social Security Act　　　　　　B. The Medicare

　　C. The Depression　　　　　　　　　　D. The Internet

3. In _____, penicillin becomes widely used.

　　A. 1930s　　　　　　B. 1940s　　　　　　C. 1950s　　　　　　D. 1960s

4. The price of hospital care _____ because of all the new services.

　　A. increased　　　　B. decreased　　　　C. tripled　　　　D. doubled

5. By 2010, _____ revolutionize communication.

　　A. The Internet　　　B. Twitter　　　C. WebMD　　　D. Social networking sites

🗒 Words and Phrases

penicillin /penɪˈsɪlɪn/ n. 盘尼西林(青霉素)

glaucoma /ɡlɔːˈkəʊmə/ n. [眼科]青光眼

arthritis /ɑːˈθraitis/ n. [外科]关节炎

dreaded /ˈdredid/ adj. 令人畏惧的；可怕的

inflation /ɪnˈfleɪʃ(ə)n/ n. 通货膨胀

cutting-edge /ˌkʌtɪŋ ˈedʒ/ adj. 先进的；尖端的

---

① 视频详见网站:https://pan-yz.cldisk.com/external/m/file/1055138526060044288。

Part II Read to Explore Medical Knowledge

Text A

Pre-reading Questions:

1. What do you know about the U.S. health care system?

2. How do you define an effective health care system?

Is the American Health Care System on Track to Overtake All Others in the World?

Text A

1. Surprisingly little data backs up the widespread opinion among Americans that our health care system is the best in the world. Conversely, since 2004, assessments published by the Commonwealth Fund have repeatedly placed the United States' health care system worst among high-income nations, even though our country spends a lot more money on health care than these other nations. These reports, which are based on data on health outcomes collected by international organizations and recent surveys of primary care physicians and the general public by the Commonwealth Fund, highlight a number of reasons why, despite providing some of the most specialized and technologically sophisticated treatments available, the U. S. health care falls short of other high-income countries' health care systems. Gaining insight into these causes could lead to crucial advancements.

2. The goal of a high-performing health care system is to deliver care that improves the health of individuals and populations. The population of the United States is sicker and dies at a higher rate than that of other high-income nations, which presents a difficulty. The United States has a considerably higher death rate from conditions that can be efficiently controlled

and treated than other high-income countries, a phenomenon known as "mortality amenable to health care," despite the fact that health care systems are not able to cure every illness. Moreover, the United States' progress in lowering that mortality has lagged behind other nations.

3. The key strategies for improving the health of a country's population through health care are to promote timely access to preventive, acute, and chronic care and to deliver evidence-based and appropriate care services. Timely access for people at risk for poor health may be impeded by three features of health care systems: the cost of care and its affordability for individuals, the administrative burden (or hassle) that people confront as they obtain and receive care, and disparities or inequities in the delivery of care based on income, educational attainment, race or ethnic background, or other nonclinical personal characteristics. Expense, administrative strain and disparities all discourage patients from seeking or retaining care. Moreover, because of their lower wealth, poorer educational background or minority status, these three characteristics have a disproportionately negative impact on the quality of care for groups with higher health risks. Consequently, other essential components of a high-performing health care system include offering sufficient insurance and minimizing administrative load and service inequities.

4. The Commonwealth Fund publications point out a number of ways that the American health care system falls short of putting these strategies into practice. Patients and physicians report that our system performs poorly in terms of administrative efficiency and timely and affordable access to care. Compared to other nations, it also has more income-related differences in care quality and access. Positively, the United States performs on equal or even better role than other nations in a number of patient-centered care processes, and on disease-specific outcomes for acute myocardial infarction, ischemic stroke, colon cancer, and breast cancer.

5. Lack of access to health care is the first problem the American health care system has to deal with. The United Kingdom, Australia, and the Netherlands are high-income nations that rank highest in the most current Fund report. They provide universal insurance coverage with low out-of-pocket expenses for preventive and primary care. Affordable and comprehensive insurance coverage is fundamental. If people are uninsured, some delay

seeking care, some of those end up with serious health problems, and some of them pass away.

6. The other problem is, in comparison to other nations, the underinvestment in primary care in the United States. Primary care is more extensively and consistently supplied in other nations. In contrast to the United States, a higher percentage of these countries' professional workforce is dedicated to primary care than to specialty care, and they enable delivery of a wider range of services at first contact, even at night and on weekends.

7. The third problem is the American health care system's administrative inefficiencies. Both professionals and patients are baffled by the complexity of getting care and paying for it in the United States. Clinicians and their staff spend countless hours completing documentation to prove that insurance coverage is active, that benefits and services are covered, that services were delivered, and that payment or reimbursement occurred. Dealing with the byzantine layers of administration results in high levels of burnout for doctors and other professionals, which can reduce the quality of care. Patients are also impacted by the complexity; they frequently receive unclear benefit descriptions, little information on physicians and hospitals, incomprehensible and frequently unexpected (or "surprise") bills for treatments, and variable copayments at lab and pharmacy. By simplifying our reimbursement systems to employ global payments, fee schedules, formularies, and defined benefits, we can lower the complexity that stands in the way of patients' and clinicians' adherence and follow-up. This would increase patient and clinician profit predictability and make benefits and costs more predictable for patients.

8. The fourth problem is the pervasiveness in the United States of disparities in the delivery of care. In all nations, but especially in the U.S., where there is a less robust social safety net than in other high-income nations, people with low incomes, low educational attainment, and other social and economic difficulties are more likely to have health problems and worse health. Other nations with healthier populations do so by spending a comparatively larger portion of their budget on social services than on health care. The need for emergency, hospital, and long-term care services may decline if resources are allocated through social spending to stable housing, educational opportunities, nutrition, and transportation in addition to ensuring that primary care is widely available and accessible to

the impoverished.

9. By launching coordinated efforts to address each of these problems, the U.S. might have the greatest-performing health care system in the world. The health of the American people might be greatly enhanced by ensuring universal and sufficient health insurance coverage, enhancing primary care, lowering administrative costs, and minimizing income-related gaps by enhancing social service and mental health programs. These fundamental adjustments could ensure that people are better equipped to manage their own health, promote prevention, reduce delayed diagnosis and treatment, and decrease ineffective or delayed diagnosis. These advancements would not only lower mortality that is treatable with medical care, but they may also, in the long run, decrease the need for extremely costly acute care "rescue" services, which would save costs.

10. The U.S. politicians have been locked in a partisan debate over dramatic legislative options for federal health care reform ranging from adoption of a single government payer, at one extreme, to curtailing federal involvement in health care, at the other. A distinctly American path for improving the U.S. health care has already been defined by two significant health care reforms: the bipartisan Medicare Access and CHIP Reauthorization Act (MACRA) of 2015 and the Affordable Care Act (ACA) of 2010. Millions of people have gained affordable insurance coverage and access to care under the ACA, and more could gain coverage through further Medicaid expansion and stabilization of individual insurance markets. Moreover, the ACA strengthened the Centers for Medicare and Medicaid Services' ability to push for payment reforms that support primary care.

11. Reversing the ACA's progress is unlikely to help the United States perform at the highest level, considering the magnitude of the issues mentioned above. There are important lessons to be learned from other affluent nations on controlling the escalating costs of health care, reforming the primary care workforce of the future, innovating to lower administrative burden and complexity, and minimizing inequities. Rather than going backward, the United States could become the first high-income nation and enhance the health of its citizens by tackling all four challenges with new laws and renewed commitments from payers, providers, and regulators.

✍ New Words and Expressions

New Words and Expressions

amendable /əˈmendəbl/ *adj.* an flaw capable of being corrected by additions 改善的

impede /ɪmˈpiːd/ *v.* (formal) to delay or stop the progress of sth. 阻碍；阻止

affordability /əˌfɔːrdəˈbɪlɪti/ *n.* the ability to pay 可购性；负担能力

hassle /ˈhæsl/ *n.* a situation that is annoying because it involves doing sth. difficult or complicated that needs a lot of effort 困难；麻烦

disparity /dɪˈspærəti/ *n.* (formal) a difference, especially one connected with unfair treatment(尤指因不公正对待引起的)不同；不等；差异；悬殊

disproportionately /dɪsprəˈpɔːʃənətli/ *adv.* not in proportion 不成比例地

myocardial /ˌmaɪəʊˈkɑːdɪəl/ *adj.* of or relating to the muscular tissue of the heart 心肌的

infarction /ɪnˈfɑːkʃn/ *n.* (medical 医) a condition in which the blood supply to an area of tissue is blocked and the tissue dies 梗塞；梗死

colon /ˈkəʊlən/ *n.* the part of the large intestine between the cecum and the rectum; it extracts moisture from food residues before they are excreted 结肠

preventive /prɪˈventɪv/ *adj.* intended to try to stop sth. that causes problems or difficulties from happening 预防性的；防备的

underinvestment /ˈʌndəɪnˈvestmənt/ *n.* an insufficient in investment 投资不足

dedicated /ˈdedɪkeɪtɪd/ *adj.* ~ (to sth.) working hard at sth. because it is very important to you 献身的；专心致志的；一心一意的

baffle /ˈbæfl/ *v.* to confuse sb. completely; to be too difficult or strange for sb. to understand or explain 使困惑；难住

byzantine /baɪˈzæntaɪn/ *adj.* 1. connected with Byzantium or the Eastern Roman Empire 拜占庭帝国的；东罗马帝国的 2. (also byzantine) (formal) (of an idea, a system, etc.) complicated, secret and difficult to change (思想、制度等)复杂神秘而死板的

burnout /ˈbɜːnaʊt/ *n.* the state of being extremely tired or ill, either physically or mentally, because you have worked too hard 精疲力竭；过度劳累

formulary /ˈfɔːmjʊlərɪ/ n. a book or system of prescribed formulas, esp. relating to religious procedure or doctrine (尤指宗教程序或教条的)公式集；配方书

pervasiveness /pəˈveisivnəs/ n. the quality of filling or spreading throughout 到处都是的状态

robust /rəʊˈbʌst/ adj. 1. strong and healthy (of a system or an organization) 强健的；强壮的(体制或机构)；2. strong and not likely to fail or become weak 强劲的；富有活力的

partisan /ˌpɑːtɪˈzæn/ adj. showing too much support for one person, group or idea, especially without considering it carefully(对某个人、团体或思想)过分支持的；偏护的；盲目拥护的

bipartisan /ˌbaɪpɑːtɪˈzæn/ adj. involving two political parties 两党的；涉及两党的

stabilization /ˌsteɪbəlaɪˈzeɪʃn/ n. the state of being stable 稳定性

📋 Notes

1. the Commonwealth Fund：It is a private foundation that aims to promote a high performing health care system that achieves better access, improved quality, and greater efficiency, particularly for society's most vulnerable, including low-income people, the uninsured, minority Americans, young children, and elderly adults.

联邦基金是一个私立基金,其目的是推动建立一个高效的医疗保障系统、为社会中最弱势的群体(包括低收入人群、无医疗保障的人群、美国少数族裔、年幼儿童以及老年人)获得医疗保障提供更好的渠道、更高的质量以及更高的效率。

2. the Patient Protection and Affordable Care Act (ACA)：The Patient Protection and Affordable Care Act, often shortened to the Affordable Care Act (ACA) or nicknamed Obamacare, is a United States federal statute enacted by the 111th United States Congress and signed into law by President Barack Obama on March 23, 2010. Together with the Health Care and Education Reconciliation Act of 2010 amendment, it represents the U.S. health care system's most significant regulatory overhaul and expansion of coverage since the passage of Medicare and Medicaid in 1965.

《患者保护与平价医疗法案》,通常缩写为 ACA,又被称为"奥巴马医保法案"。ACA 是由美国第 111 届国会签署通过的美国联邦法规,并于 2010 年 3 月 23 日由奥巴马签署生效。奥巴马医保与 2010 年的《医疗保障与教育和解法案(修正案)》共同代表了自 1965 年的联邦医疗保险和医疗补助计划后美国医疗保障体系中最重要的法规上的修复与完善以及覆盖范围上的扩大。

3. Medicare Access and CHIP Reauthorization ACT（MACRA）：On April 16, 2015, President Obama signed into law the Medicare Access and CHIP Reauthorization Act of 2015 （MACRA）.

2015 年 4 月 16 日,奥巴马总统签署了《联邦医疗保险入保和儿童健康保险计划再授权法案》。

4. Medicaid：In the United States, Medicaid is a joint federal and state program that helps with medical costs for some people with limited income and resources. Medicaid also offers benefits not normally covered by Medicare, like nursing home care and personal care services. Medicaid is the largest source of funding for medical and health-related services for people with low income in the United States, providing free health insurance to 74 million low-income and disabled people.

美国的医疗补助计划是联邦及州两级政府共同出资的补助计划,旨在帮助支付一些收入及资源不足人群的医疗花费。医疗补助计划同时也会提供联邦医疗保险没有覆盖的部分,如家庭护理及个人护理服务。医疗补助计划是美国对低收入人群所提供的最大型的医疗健康服务基金,为 7400 万低收入及残障人士提供免费的医疗保险。

5. Medicare：Medicare is a U.S. government health insurance program beginning from 1965. It is a national program that subsidizes health care services for anyone 65 or older, younger people with disabilities, and patients with end-stage renal disease. Medicare is divided into four components：Medicare Part A, Part B, Part C (also called Medicare Advantage), and Part D for prescription drugs. Medicare Part A premiums are free for those who made Medicare contributions through payroll taxes for at least 10 years. Patients are responsible for paying premiums for other parts of the Medicare program.

医疗保险是美国政府从 1965 年开始的一项健康保险计划。这是一项国家计划,为 65 岁或以上的人、年轻的残疾人和终末期肾病患者提供医疗保健服务补贴。医疗保险分为四个部分:处方药的医疗保险 A 部分、B 部分、C 部分(也被称为"医疗保险优惠")和 D 部分。对于通过工资缴纳医疗保险税至少 10 年的人来说，医疗保险 A 部分的保费是免费的。患者需要负责支付医疗保险计划其他部分(B、C 和 D)的保费。

☰ After Reading Activities

Reading Comprehension

✅ I. Answer the following questions.

1. Why does the U.S. health care system fail to achieve the level of performance of other countries?
2. What can be done to improve the health of the country's population through health care?
3. Are there any positive sides in the U.S. health care system?
4. What are the four challenges the U.S. health care system must confront?
5. What are the benefits of the two major reforms to the U.S. health care system?

✅ II. Work in groups to complete the following chart according to the structure of the text.

What is the problem：(paras. 1-2)

Reports from the Commonwealth Fund have consistently ＿＿＿＿＿＿＿＿ among high-income countries, despite the fact that we spend far more on health care than these other countries. That is to say, U.S. health care ＿＿＿＿＿＿＿＿ of other high-income countries. (Para 1)

Causes of the problem：(paras. 3-8)

The key strategies for improving the health of a country's population through health care are to promote timely access to preventive, acute, and chronic care and to deliver evidence-based and appropriate care services. However, timely access for people at risk for poor health may be impeded by three features of health care systems：＿＿＿＿＿＿＿＿ , ＿＿＿＿＿＿＿＿, ＿＿＿＿＿＿＿＿. (para. 3)

Also, the U.S. health care system confront four challenges：

First, ＿＿＿＿＿＿＿＿＿＿＿＿＿＿＿＿＿＿＿＿.

Second, ＿＿＿＿＿＿＿＿＿＿＿＿＿＿＿＿＿＿＿＿.

Third, _____.

Fourth, _____.

Solutions to the problems: (paras. 9-10)

The U.S. could achieve the best-performed health care system in the world by _____, ensuring _____, strengthening _____, lowering _____, reducing _____. (para. 9)

Conclusion: (para. 11)

Rather than going backward, the United States could become the _____ high-income nation and enhance _____ by tackling all four challenges with _____ and _____ from payers, providers, and regulators.

Words and Phrases

✅ I. Translate the following medical terms into Chinese or English.

1. health insurance coverage   _____

2. delayed diagnosis   _____

3. primary care   _____

4. specialty care   _____

5. 心肌梗死   _____

6. 缺血性脑卒中   _____

7. 结肠癌   _____

8. 预防性护理   _____

✅ II. Fill in the blanks with the words or phrases given below. Change the form if necessary.

mortality	acute	chronic	pervasiveness	preventive

1. Prostate cancer is a slow growing cancer, and if you can slow it down even further, you can turn it from a fatal condition to a _____ one that can be managed.

2. Back in the early 1990s, we never would have suspected that population growth would have turned negative because of AIDS _____.

3. This year, all new insurance plans will be required to offer free _____ care to their

customs so that we can start catching preventable illnesses and diseases on the front end.

4. In other situations, a level who transplant may be the only cure for _____ liver failure.

5. Heart failure has become one of the most _____ cardiovascular illness in the United States.

Sentence Translation

Translate the following sentences into Chinese or English.

1. The goal of a high-performing health care system is to deliver care that improves the health of individuals and populations.

_____

_____

2. The key strategies for improving the health of a country's population through health care are to promote timely access to preventive, acute, and chronic care and to deliver evidence-based and appropriate care services.

_____

_____

3. Affordable and comprehensive insurance coverage is fundamental. If people are uninsured, some delay seeking care, some of those end up with serious health problems, and some of them pass away.

_____

_____

4. 而从 2004 年开始, 联邦基金便一直将美国医疗保障体系的表现在高收入国家中排在最后, 尽管我们花在医疗保障上的钱要比其他国家多得多。

_____

_____

5. 临床医生以及其他的员工花了无数的时间去完成文件记录, 证明保险范围有效, 证明保险覆盖了补助金及各项服务, 证明病人享受到了相应的服务, 或者是证明完成了支付或报销。

_____

_____

Text B

Pre-reading Questions:

1. What do you know about Chinese health care system?

2. How can Chinese health care system improve the public health?

An Overview of the Chinese Health Care System

Text B

1. In China, the health care security system is a crucial institutional framework that contributes to the improvement of people's health and well-being as well as the preservation of social harmony and stability. The goal of creating a national medical security system is to reduce people's concerns about getting sick and getting medical care.

The Composition, Coverage, and Operational Trend of China's National Medical Security System

2. China's national medical security system is a multilevel system that consists of commercial health insurance, philanthropic donations, and medical mutual help as supplemental services, with medical aid serving as the backup and basic medical insurance (BMI) as the pillar.

3. Both residents and employees benefit from the BMI system. The resident basic medical insurance (RBMI) program is for non-working residents, and the employee basic medical insurance (EBMI) program is for working individuals. The National Healthcare Security Administration (NHSA) was founded in 2018 and has since worked to enhance the nation's health insurance program in order to better integrate RBMI. As of September 2020, more than 1.35 billion people (over 95% of China's population) are covered by one of the BMI programs, making it the world's largest health care security network. Among those covered, 337 million are covered by the EBMI, and 1.014 billion people are covered by the RBMI. The medical insurance fund is sustainable and growing. In 2019, the revenue of the national basic medical insurance fund (including maternity insurance) was CNY ￥2.44

trillion, and the expenditure was CNY ￥2.09 trillion.

4. Medical aid ensures all citizens have fair access to basic medical services by supporting the section of the low-income populace to participate in the BMI by subsidizing the medical expenses that they cannot afford. Since 2018, medical aid has benefited 480 million low-income citizens, helped reduce their medical burden by approximately CNY ￥330 billion, implemented targeted poverty reduction measures for 10 million people in need who were impoverished due to illnesses, and ensured their basic medical security. Various social forces in the market also actively participate in supplementing the medical security system and have become an important element of the multilevel medical insurance system.

Characteristics and Advantages of China's Health Care Security System

5. The Chinese government has consistently provided the BMI as a public utility for all Chinese citizens, viewing people's health and life safety as a fundamental duty. However, a deficit in coverage still exists between China and other countries with developed social security systems. The proportion of total medical insurance financing is about 2.5% of China's GDP, which is not high, but it is generally compatible with the per capita GDP of U.S. $10,000 in China.

I. Provide more. For one, government funding should be increased. From 2007 to 2019, government funding for medical security increased from CNY ￥91.3 billion to CNY ￥800 billion, and the proportion of government spending on medical insurance increased from 1.87% to 3.50%. In 2020, the government subsidy for resident medical security reached CNY ￥550 per person. For another, focus should remain on the low-income population. Policies should lean towards the low-income population to ensure they have access to the BMI. The government continued to increase funding, and more than 99.9% of registered low-income citizens are now insured. The imbursement rate of hospitalization expenses has stabilized at around 80% for the low-income population after the broad coverage provided by the triple security system: the BMI, critical illness insurance, and medical aid.

II. Stay within economic capabilities. To ensure the sustainable balance of the fund, financial overcommitment should be avoided, and the planning should be informed by the current level of economic development. The fund should meet the basic needs of people, but it should avoid becoming a welfare fund.

III. Reinforcing the administration of the security system. First, a nationally organized volume-based procurement and use of drug standard should be established. A total of 112 types of drugs were procured by China in three batches, with the costs decreasing by an average of 54%, which saved CNY ¥53.9 billion annually. Second, the catalog of medicines covered by the national health security system should be dynamically adjusted. Some obsolete drugs have been removed from the catalog to make room for drugs with more clinical value. Third, a reformation of medical insurance payment methods needs to be steadily implemented. In China, 97.5% of the local administrations have capped the total regional expense of medical insurance, and more than 30 pilot cities have launched diagnosis-related group payment systems. Fourth, medical organizations should be strictly supervised and unlawful practices should be heavily penalized. 330,000 illegal organizations have been suspended in the last two years, and CNY ¥12.56 billion in money have been recovered. During 69 inspection teams' surprise field inspections in 30 regions nationwide in 2019, illicit cash worth CNY ¥2.232 billion was discovered.

Reforming the Drug Pricing Mechanism and Promoting Drug Availability for Patients

6. The NHSA has implemented dynamic adjustments to the catalog of medicines covered by the national health security system and issued the *Interim Measures on the Administration of Medicines under the Basic Medical Insurance*. The goal of the interim measures is to ensure that drug costs are in line with BMI financing and to satisfy residents' basic medical needs. Ensuring a medical insurance medication management system that is exact, standardized, dynamic, and scientific is vital. Negotiation based on catalog access determines the price of exclusively produced drugs, saving medical insurance money while also drastically lowering the cost to patients. The prompt addition of more efficacious medications to the inventory may be facilitated by the implementation of a dynamic adjustment mechanism.

7. The administration of medications related to hepatitis is a good example of this. Thanks to the government's persistent efforts, the cost of medications treating viral hepatitis has significantly decreased in recent years. In 2015, the annual treatment cost of hepatitis B antiviral drugs, tenofovir disoproxil fumarate (TDF) and entecavir, was about CNY

¥9,000 and CNY ¥20,000 per person, respectively. In 2018, after the "4+7" Pilot Program was launched, the annual treatment cost of TDF and entecavir was decreased to CNY ¥210 to 240 per person. In 2019, after more cities were included in the pilot program, the cost of the two drugs was further decreased to CNY ¥70. After the centralized procurement of entecavir, the total procurement volume was 3.5 times lower than that of the previous year in the "4+7" pilot cities. In the same year, a number of oral hepatitis C medications were negotiated and reimbursed by the NHSA, resulting in a 95% decrease in patient out-of-pocket costs. The World Health Organization's 2030 Sustainable Development Goal—eliminating hepatitis as a threat to public health—was made possible in China by the significant drop in drug prices, which also led to improvements in the diagnosis rate and accessibility of chronic hepatitis treatment.

Building A Multilevel Medical Security System to Reinforce Support Capabilities

8. In recent years, China's commercial health insurance premium income has developed rapidly at an annual growth rate of 30%. Commercial health insurance premium income in 2019 was CNY ¥706.6 billion, a 29.7% rise from the previous year. The government suggests strengthening the triple security system—which consists of basic medical insurance, critical illness insurance, and medical aid—as well as promoting a number of supplemental medical insurance programs for major and critical diseases in order to address the rising demand for health care in the modern era. There will be an acceleration of the development of commercial health insurance, an increase in the number of health insurance products available, a more efficient application of the individual income tax policies pertaining to commercial health insurance, and a greater range of insurance products.

Seizing Opportunities, Meeting Challenges, and Promoting the High-Quality Development of Medical Security

9. The year 2020 is the final year of the *13th Five-Year Plan*, and it is also the year to lay a good foundation for the *14th Five-Year Plan*. Standing at this critical juncture, it is necessary to have a clear understanding of the challenges faced by health security.

10. The demographics of the Chinese population poses serious challenges to the sustainability of the fund. By the time the *14th Five-Year Plan* ends, there will be more than 300 million

adults over the age of 60, and the proportion of working age people to retirees will keep falling. The "double burden" that chronic illnesses and communicable diseases place on China's medical insurance budget is another significant obstacle. The expectations of citizens regarding medical care and the support provided by health care security still differ.

11. Medical security is highly relevant to the vital interests of the Chinese people as a whole. During the *14th Five-Year Plan* period, the government will continue to support the integrity of the multilevel medical security and direct the coordinated development of medical security, treatment, and medicine in order to have more realistic expectations for public health security and, consequently, a greater sense of gain, healthy security, and happiness for the public.

New Words and Expressions

New Words and
Expressions

composition /ˌkɒmpəˈzɪʃn/ *n.* a mixture of ingredients 组成；成分

multilevel /ˌmʌltɪˈlɛvl/ *adj.* of a building having more than one level 多层次的

maternity /məˈtɜːnəti/ *n.* the state of being or becoming a mother 母亲身份；怀孕；产科；*adj.*用法

populace /ˈpɒpjələs/ *n.* (formal) all the ordinary people of a particular country or area 平民百姓；民众；人口

subsidize /ˈsʌbsɪdaɪz/ *v.* to give money to sb. or an organization to help pay for sth.; to give a subsidy 资助；补助；给……发津贴

approximately /əˈprɒksɪmətli/ *adv.* used to show that sth. is almost, but not completely, accurate or correct 大概；大约

impoverish /ɪmˈpɒvərɪʃ/ *v.* make sb. poor; to make sth. worse in quality 使贫穷；使贫瘠；使枯竭

deficit /ˈdefɪsɪt/ *n.* the amount by which sth., especially an amount of money, is too small or smaller than sth. else 不足额；缺款额；赤字

subsidy /ˈsʌbsədi/ *n.* money that is paid by a government or an organization to reduce the costs of services or of producing goods so that their prices can be kept low 补贴；补助金；津贴；资助

imbursement /ɪmˈbɜːsmənt/ *n.* similar to "reimbursement", and it refers to the act of reimbursing or compensating someone for expenses, losses, or services rendered. It is the process of paying back money that was spent by an individual on behalf of someone else or for a particular purpose 支付；报销

reinforce /ˌriːɪnˈfɔːs/ *v.* to make a feeling, an idea, etc. stronger 加强；充实；使更强烈；加固

procurement /prəˈkjuəmənt/ *n.* (formal) the process of obtaining supplies of sth., especially for a government or an organization (尤指为政府或机构) 采购；购买

catalog /ˈkætəlɒg/ *n.* a complete list of items, for example of things that people can look at or buy 目录；目录簿

obsolete /ˈɒbsəliːt/ *adj.* no longer used because sth. new has been invented 过时的；陈旧的

cap /kæp/ *v.* (especially BrE) to limit the amount of money that can be charged for sth. or spent on sth. 限额收取(或支出)

penalize /ˈpiːnəlaɪz/ *v.* ~ sb. (for sth.) to punish sb. for breaking a rule or law by making them suffer a disadvantage 处罚；惩罚；处以刑罚

interim /ˈɪntərɪm/ *adj.* intended to last for only a short time until sb. /sth. more permanent is found 暂时的；过渡的

hepatitis /ˌhepəˈtaɪtɪs/ *n.* a serious disease of the liver 肝炎

antiviral /ˌænti ˈvaɪrəl/ *adj.* used to treat infectious diseases caused by a virus 抗病毒的

entecavir /entɪkæˈvɜː/ *n.* abbreviated ETV, is an oral antiviral drug used in the treatment of hepatitis B virus (HBV) infection 恩替卡韦(一种抗病毒药物)

premium /ˈpriːmiəm/ *n.* an amount of money that you pay once or regularly for an insurance policy 保险费

juncture /ˈdʒʌŋktʃə(r)/ *n.* (formal) a particular point or stage in an activity or a series of events 特定时刻；关头

demographics /ˌdeməˈgræfɪks/ *n.* (statistics 统计) data relating to the population and different groups within it 人口统计数据；人口特征

sustainability /səsˌteɪnəˈbɪlɪti/ *n.* the property of being sustainable 可持续性；可维持性

📑 Notes

1. BMI：It refers to basic medical insurance. 基本医疗保险。

2. EBMI：It refers to employee basic medical insurance (EBMI). 职工基本医疗保险。

3. RBMI：It refers to residents' basic medical insurance. More than 95 percent of Chinese were covered by the country's national basic medical insurance programs in 2019.

居民基本医疗保险。2019 年，全国居民基本医疗保险参保率超过 95%。

4. NHSA：National Health and Security Administration 国家医疗保障局

5. TDF：Tenofovir disoproxil fumarate (TDF), a novel nucleotide reverse transcriptase inhibitor (NRTI), was used in patients with HIV co-infected with HBV. And it is still a vital first-line antiretroviral compounds in HAART.

富马酸替诺福韦二吡呋酯(TDF)是一种新型核苷酸逆转录酶抑制剂(NRTI)，用于 HIV 合并 HBV 感染的患者。它是 HAART 中重要的一线抗逆转录病毒化合物。

6. "4+7" Pilot Program：A new VBP pilot (i. e., the "4+7" pilot) program in China was introduced in December 2018 and officially launched in March 2019. Under this VBP, the Chinese government centralizes the purchasing process nationwide and pre-defines the purchase quantity. Manufacturers compete on price by submitting bids.

2018 年 12 月，中国启动了新的药品集中采购试点(即"4+7"试点)，并于 2019 年 3 月正式启动。在这种机制下，中国政府在全国范围内集中采购过程，并预先确定采购数量。制造商通过投标进行价格竞争。

📄 After Reading Activities

Reading Comprehension

Decide whether the following statements are true (T) or false (F) according to the text.

_____ 1. The aim of establishing a national medical security system is to relieve all people of their worries about illness and health care.

_____ 2. The national medical security system in China is a multilevel system, with the basic medical insurance (BMI) as the backup and medical aid as the pillar, and commercial health insurance, charitable donations, and medical mutual aid activities as main services.

_____ 3. To ensure the sustainable balance of the fund, financial overcommitment should be avoided, and the planning should be informed by the current level of economic development. The fund of health care should be the more the better.

_____ 4. To meet people's growing needs of health care in the new era, the government proposes to strengthen the triple security system, including basic medical insurance, critical illness insurance, and medical aid, and promote various complementary medical insurance programs for major and critical diseases.

_____ 5. The health care security support in China can fully meet the medical expectations of citizens already.

Words and Phrases

Match each English phrase in Column A with its Chinese version in Column B.

Column A	Column B
1. health care security system	A. 独家专利生产药物
2. social harmony and stability	B. 医疗保障体系
3. maternity insurance	C. 个人所得税政策
4. targeted poverty reduction	D. 社会和谐和稳定
5. volume-based procurement	E. 自付费用
6. exclusively produced drugs	F. 药品集中带量采购
7. out-of-pocket cost	G. 精准扶贫
8. individual income tax policies	H. 生育保险

Translation

目前，中国共有三种医疗保险政策：一种是1998年建立的城镇职工保险制度，另一种是2003年建立的新型农村合作医疗制度，还有一种就是2007年建立的城镇居民医疗制度。其中，后两者是政府大力补助的，而城镇职工保险制度，是由员工和雇主共同支付费用，有着最佳的偿还率。

_____

_____

_____

_____

Critical Thinking

Can you make a comparison of the health care system between China and the U.S. according to what you have learned from our texts?

Part III　Apply Medical English

Dialogue

A. Situational Dialogues while Receiving a Patient from Other Countries

Registration(分诊)

Nurse: Hello, I am Nurse Li Dehong. My English name is Linda. Please call me Nurse Linda. Can I help you?

Patient: I want to see a doctor. I'm ill.

Nurse: What are your symptoms?

Patient: I have been experiencing diarrhea and vomiting for the last couple of days.

Nurse: You need to see a doctor in the Emergency Room. Do you understand Chinese?

Patient: Not at all.

Nurse: You need to register first and then see the emergency doctor. I will take you to the Emergency Department. Would you like a wheelchair? The registration fee is 7 yuan. Please wait a moment, and I will get a form for you.

Patient: Thank you.

Nurse: Here is the registration form, and you will need to write the answers to a few questions. What is your name?

Patient: Paula Jones.

Nurse: What is your date of birth?

Patient: 8. 9. 1963.

Nurse: Is that 8th, September 1963 or 9th, August 1963?

Patient: 8th, September 1963.

Nurse: What is your address here in Beijing?

Patient: Hotel Beijing, Wangfujing.

Nurse: Are you a tourist?

Patient: Yes, I am.

Nurse: Can I have your address in your own country, please?

Patient: 16a, Crowthorne Crescent, Handscross, West Sussex, BN12 7RN.

Nurse: Please can you write that down on this form for me? What is your nationality?

Patient: Yes, of course. I'm British.

Nurse: What is your telephone number?

Patient: My mobile number is 7079857432.

Nurse: Who is your next of kin?

Patient: Mr. David Jones.

Nurse: Can you write his name and address and telephone number, please?

Patient: Yes, certainly.

Nurse: Do you have health insurance?

Patient: Yes, I do.

Nurse: Even though you have health insurance, you will have to pay the medical bill first and then claim. You will receive a letter from the hospital to submit your insurance claim.

Patient: OK, I see.

Nurse: In your case, you will have to pay your medical bill before you leave the hospital.

Patient: OK.

Nurse: I will take this form back to the counter and get your paperwork. Can I have 7 yuan for the registration fee, please? Please stay here, and I will come back.

Patient: Thank you.

Nurse: I will guide you to the ER doctor now.

Patient: Thank you.

Nurse: Is there anything else I can do for you?

Patient: No, thanks. You've been very kind.

Nurse: You are welcome. I hope you get better soon. Goodbye.

Words and Phrases

vomiting /ˈvɒmɪtɪŋ/ v. 呕吐

wheelchair /ˈwiːltʃeə(r)/ n. 轮椅

next of kin /ˌnekst əv ˈkɪn/ 近亲

medical bill /ˈmedɪkl bɪl/ 医药费

claim /kleɪm/ v. 索要；索取

⊞ Notes

Some reminders for foreigners to receive medical service in China

1. Preparing Necessary Documents and Procedures

First, foreigners need to provide a valid passport and visa to ensure their legal stay in China. Additionally, to benefit from medical insurance, they must present proof of medical insurance in China. Medical insurance is crucial for covering medical expenses, so foreigners should ensure they have purchased and hold valid insurance before seeking medical care.

2. Choosing an Appropriate Medical Facility

Selecting the right medical facility is an important task for foreigners. It is advisable to prioritize accredited medical institutions to ensure quality and safety of treatment. Some hospitals may have special windows or reception areas specifically for foreigners to offer more personalized services.

3. Registration Procedures

Before receiving medical care, foreigners need to go to the hospital for registration. Typically, they need to provide their passport, visa, medical insurance proof, and contact information. Some hospitals might require additional forms to be filled out or additional identification documents for record-keeping.

4. Payment and Reimbursement Matters

During the medical visit, foreigners should understand and adhere to the hospital's payment and reimbursement policies. Generally, foreigners in China need to bear part of the medical expenses themselves, especially at private clinics or non-insurance designated hospitals. However, with valid medical insurance, foreigners can apply for partial reimbursement from the insurance company after treatment. Therefore, before seeking medical care, they should consult with their insurance company about the relevant policies and prepare the necessary documents.

5. Compliance with Relevant Policies and Regulations

Foreigners must comply with relevant policies and regulations when seeking medical care in China to ensure the process is legal and compliant. Firstly, they must abide by Chinese laws and regulations during their stay, including entry and exit management, public security management, and visa extensions. Secondly, they must adhere to China's medical and health management regulations, medical insurance policies, and other relevant laws when receiving medical care.

6. Other Considerations

During medical treatment, foreigners should also be mindful of other considerations, such as medical confidentiality agreements and emergency rescue protocols. Additionally, some hospitals may require foreigners to provide relevant medical history or undergo certain examinations before treatment to better develop a treatment plan.

外国人在中国就医须知：

一、准备必要的文件和手续

首先，外国人需要提供有效的护照和签证，以确保其在中国的合法逗留。同时，为了享受医疗保险，外国人还需提供在华的医疗保险证明。在中国，医疗保险是医疗费用报销的重要保障，因此外国人在就医前应确保已购买并持有有效的医疗保险。

二、选择合适的医疗机构

对于外国人来说，选择合适的医疗机构是一项重要任务。在选择医院时，建议优先考虑正规医疗机构，以确保治疗质量和安全。对于外籍人士，部分医院可能会特别设置专门的窗口或接待处，以便为他们提供更个性化的服务。

三、挂号和登记手续

就医前，外国人需要前往医院挂号并登记。通常，外国人需要提供护照、签证、医疗保险证明以及联系方式等相关信息。部分医院可能会要求外国人填写额外的表格或提供身份证明文件以供存档。

四、支付和报销事宜

在就医过程中，外国人需要了解并遵守医院的支付和报销政策。通常，外国人在中国就医时需要自行承担部分医疗费用，尤其是私人诊所或非医保定点医院。然而，在持有有效医疗保险的情况下，外国人可以在就医后向保险公司申请报销部分医疗费用。因此，在就医前，外国人应向保险公司咨询相关政策并备齐所需文件。

五、遵守相关政策和法规

外国人在中国就医时需要遵守相关政策和法规，以确保就医过程合法合规。首先，外国人在华逗留期间必须遵守中国的法律和规定，包括出入境管理、治安管理、签证延期等方面的规定。其次，外国人在中国就医时必须遵守中国的医疗卫生管理条例、医疗保险政策等相关法规。

六、其他注意事项

在就医过程中，外国人还需注意其他一些事项，如医疗保密协议、紧急救援等方面的规定。此外，部分医院可能会要求外国人在就医前提供相关病史资料或进行相关检查，以便更好地制定治疗方案。

Practical Activity

Work with your partner to create and perform a nurse-patient dialogue related to filling the registration form, including following information: name, date of birth, address (Chinese address and home country address), nationality, passport number, telephone number, medical insurance number, etc..

Guidance for
Production

B. Practical Unit Project

You can compose your own essay (150-200 words) by learning the following opinions, and pick up YES or NO.

Should the government make sure that every American has affordable health insurance?	
YES	NO
• Health care is a right and as a matter of social justice the government should be responsible for making sure that every American has access to affordable coverage and quality care.	• Creating a guarantee of universal coverage would vastly expand the role of the federal government in the lives of the American people, who are better off with the freedom to make their own health care choices.
• Expanding eligibility for government programs like Medicare and Medicaid could cover large ranks of the uninsured.	• Large government programs are almost always inefficient and broadening eligibility would increase federal spending dramatically.
• Increased government regulation could prevent health insurers from rejecting anyone for coverage because of preexisting conditions or basing rates on their health.	• Regulatory mandates will increase costs, which insurance companies will pass along to consumers.
• Government provided health insurance would compete with private plans on cost and would reduce the number of Americans who are uninsured and underinsured.	• A public plan would have a competitive advantage that will drive private plans out of business, leaving consumers with no choice.

Tips for writing an opinion or argumentative essay:

Part 1：An introduction

Introduce the central message of your essay.

Part 2：Background of the subject

Introduce early studies about your topic.

Part 3：Main arguments

Talk about the main points of your position. Use examples, figures, evidences to support your point.

Part 4：Refutation

Here is where your counterarguments come into place. Introduce the opposite side you will need to refute as being invalid. Give more statistics and evidences would be helpful to make your essay more convincing.

Part 5：Conclusion

Present all of the main arguments and provide solutions or studies that need to be concluded in the future.

Part IV   Self-Assessment

Use the following self-assessment checklist to check what you have learned in this unit.

I understand the basic concept and structure of health care system in the U.S..	☐
I can identify and use the words, phrases and sentence patterns related to the topic.	☐
I can write an essay about how to confront challenges of health care system in the U.S. by using the terminologies and medical information in this unit.	☐
I can compare and understand the differences of health care system between China and the U.S..	☐

Unit 4
Traditional Chinese Medicine

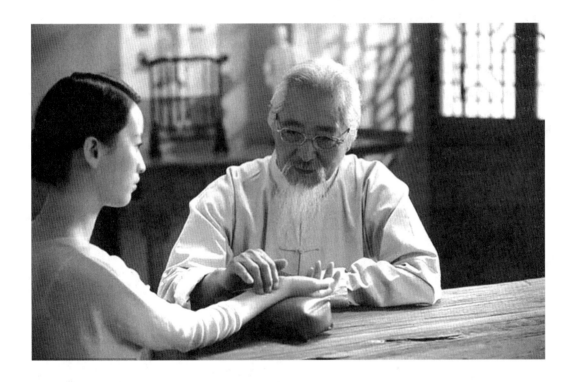

Traditional Chinese Medicine（中医）, also called "TCM", is an ancient system of traditional medicine developed in China over thousands of years. Although seeking TCM treatment is still somewhat uncommon in the West, it's hard to spend much time in China without realizing that TCM still enjoys a booming popularity there.

Walk down any street and you're likely to bump into several pharmacies selling traditional Chinese herbal medicines. You're also likely to hear Chinese people make frequent reference to TCM-related concepts, like the idea that certain

Lead in

foods are "hot" while others are "cold." Chinese doctors and dentists practicing Western medicine in mainstream hospitals and clinics may even make TCM-inspired recommendations, focusing on the implementation of certain daily living habits in order to encourage well-being. Given the continued prevalence of TCM in everyday Chinese life, gaining some familiarity with it is a good idea for students. Read on to learn more about the past, present, and future of traditional Chinese medicine!

This unit is mainly to achieve the following objectives:

1) Understand the basic concept of TCM;

2) Identify words, phrases and sentence patterns related to the topic;

3) Do the translation and make a presentation by using the terminologies and medical information of TCM;

4) Spread Chinese TCM to the world and make the whole world know more about TCM.

Part I　View the Medical World

Watch a video about acupuncture and choose the right answer. ①

1. Acupuncture is the procedure has been around _____ years?

　　A. 2,400　　　　　B. 2,500　　　　　C. 250　　　　　D. 240

2. According to the video, the ancient Chinese believed that the human body had a network of life force in it, known as qi. They aim to heal the body by manipulating this qi with the aid of _____.

　　A. needles　　　　B. medicine　　　　C. acupoint　　　　D. Tuina

3. According to the video, acupuncture is believed to help with the following except _____.

　　A. strokes　　　　　　　　　　　B. PMS

　　C. homesickness　　　　　　　　D. high blood pressure

4. Which of the following is not mentioned as the advantages of acupuncture treatment?

　　A. It is quite easy to find an acupuncturist.

　　B. The sessions are not very long.

　　C. The sessions are relatively inexpensive.

　　D. You need a session every day.

5. If there is no acupuncturist in your city, or you cannot get a session, it is advisable to _____.

　　A. try it by yourself

　　B. ask your friend to help

　　C. plan a trip to a nearby city to see another acupuncturist

　　D. eat some alternative medicines by yourself

---

①　视频详见网站:https://pan-yz. cldisk. com/external/m/file/1055138561317367808。

📑 Words and Phrases

swear /sweə(r)/ v. 宣誓证明

metaphysical /ˌmetəˈfɪzɪkl/ adj. 玄学的；形而上学的

stimulate /ˈstɪmjuleɪt/ v. 鼓励；刺激

stroke /strəʊk/ n. 中风

allergy /ˈælədʒɪ/ n. 过敏

hypertension /ˌhaɪpəˈtenʃn/ n. 高血压

insomnia /ɪnˈsɒmnɪə/ n. 失眠(症)

osteoarthritis /ˌɒstiəʊɑːˈθraɪtɪs/ n. 骨关节炎

chronic pain /ˈkrɒnɪk peɪn/ 慢性疼痛

menstrual cramps/ˈmenstruəl kræmps/ 月经痛

PMS：an abbreviation for premenstrual syndrome 经前期综合征

migraine /ˈmiːgreɪn/ n. 偏头痛

sprain /spreɪn/ v./n. 关节扭伤

morning sickness /ˈmɔːnɪŋ sɪknəs/ 孕吐

Part II   Read to Explore Medical Knowledge

Text A

Pre-reading Questions:

1. What do you know about acupuncture?
2. Will you try acupuncture in medical treatment? Why and why not?

Acupuncture

Text A

1. A civilization of almost 1.4 billion people relies on Traditional Chinese Medicine (TCM), which is the cornerstone of Chinese people and has been practiced continuously for 5,000 years. Acupuncture is included as part of its medical regimen in TCM.

2. During an acupuncture treatment, sterile, disposable needles with rounded tips are inserted into certain bodily acupoints to elicit a healing response. The procedure is pain-free.

3. So, how does it work? The ancient Chinese held the view that all living things contain qi, or universal life energy (pronounced "chee"). It is believed that this energy travels through the body via particular channels known as meridians or vessels. Health is preserved as long as this energy is allowed to freely move through the meridians; but, as soon as this energy flow is obstructed, the system becomes unstable, leading to discomfort and dysfunction. Imagine electrical grid short circuits resulting in blackouts or rivers that overflow and cause calamities. Acupuncture stimulates specific meridians points to free up qi energy, which then helps to reprogram and restore normal function.

Helping to Call the Right Neurochemicals and Hormones

4. A research paper from 1999 that was published in the *American Journal of Physiology*

linked acupuncture to the release of endorphins, which are neurochemicals. In order to lower high blood pressure, the patients were given an injection by the scientists that prevents the release of endorphins before they received acupuncture. The patients who did not receive the injection experienced a significant drop in their high blood pressure, indicating a possible relationship between endorphin release and acupuncture.

5. Pain is a sign that there is a problem within the body. When it comes to pain relief, most individuals seek out acupuncture and Chinese medicine for knee pain, back pain, headaches, menstrual pain, or any other type of discomfort. This usually occurs when a disease or injury is causing poor blood flow or impaired nerve transmission. Depending on the underlying causes, a healthy body will react differently to heal the issues and reduce discomfort.

6. In order to speed up this process and help the body heal and subdue pain more quickly than it would if treatment is not received, acupuncture is used.

7. It has been shown that acupuncture modulates nerve impulses and corrects misfiring nerves in the damaged or diseased area, allowing the brain to communicate with the body properly and releasing endorphins and enkephalins, which reduce pain and naturally occur anti-inflammatory proteins. Acupuncture's process of nerve retraining guarantees that the body's healing processes perform as intended, resulting in the restoration of normal, healthy function and long-lasting pain alleviation.

Helping to Get Blood to Circulate

8. As it well known that it is all in your blood to keep you alive. Food, oxygen, hormones, medicine, and substances that stave off infection and aid in healing are all found in your blood. Longevity and optimal health are dependent on the blood traveling to the right places in your body and staying there. The Chinese proverb puts it this way: Where there is stagnation there is disease, where there is disease there is stagnation. The majority of diseases and injuries can manifest if these essential compounds are not delivered to their intended location.

9. It has been discovered that acupuncture works incredibly well to increase blood flow. Numerous studies have shown that acupuncture can increase vital blood flow to the body's deprived areas by stimulating the production of specific chemicals, including nitric oxide, leukotrienes, and antihistamines, which dilate blood vessels and reduce tissue swelling.

Being Beneficial for Severe Heart Failure

10. According to Chinese medicine, heart failure and chest pain have distinct causes. Blockage of the blood and qi circulation is the primary cause of chest pain. This barrier is brought on by deficient patterns, which include weak blood circulation and excessive viscosity (thickness). Pathogenic elements such as cholesterol or blood clots that obstruct blood circulation and qi are examples of excess patterns.

11. Studies have indicated that acupuncture may be helpful for patients experiencing severe heart failure. Acupuncture lowers activity in the sympathetic nervous system, which controls involuntary movements like blood pressure and heartbeat, by lowering the pressure on the heart. According to research conducted in Scandinavia, acupuncture can improve the heart's ability to pump blood, which can lessen pain and the need for prescription drugs.

Being Helpful for Knee Arthritis

12. A 2004 study financed by the National Institutes of Health revealed that acupuncture was effective in relieving pain associated with knee arthritis among its 570 participants, making it the largest study of its kind. "These results also indicate that acupuncture can serve as an effective addition to a standard regimen of care and improve quality of life for patients with knee osteoarthritis," stated author Stephen Straus, director of the National Center for Complementary and Alternative Medicine (NCCAM), in reference to the study. Applying stringent research methodologies to traditional practices such as acupuncture is showing great potential and power, as demonstrated by the portfolio of basic and clinical research that NCCAM has been accumulating.

Being Helpful for Increasing Fertility

13. In conjunction with in vitro fertilization (IVF), it could potentially improve the chances of successful female conception. A well-known study that appeared in the April 2002 issue of *Fertility* & *Sterility* revealed that over 40% of individuals who had acupuncture during an IVF round were able to conceive, as opposed to 26% of pregnant patients who did not undergo the therapy. Because of these success rates, many reproductive endocrinologists advise their patients who are considering fertility to add acupuncture to their treatment regimen. For as long as IVF has been an option for treatment in California, Tao of Wellness has been providing fertility medicine.

Being Helpful for Children with Chronic Pain in Pediatric Acupuncture

14. In order to help kids manage chronic pain, Yo San University of Traditional Chinese Medicine—founded by the same people who founded Tao of Wellness—collaborates with the Pediatric Pain Management Clinic at Children's Hospital Los Angeles (CHLA) to offer a pediatric acupuncture project. Drs. Daoshing and Mao Shing Ni, Wendy Yu, and Brandon Horn, as well as Dr. Jeffrey Gold, the director of the pediatric pain management clinic, started the collaboration. Yo San University interns get the chance to gain clinical experience at CHLA, a teaching hospital affiliated with University of Southern California, as part of this program.

15. In the conclusion of a paper published in the journal Evidence-Based Complementary and Alternative Medicine, Dr. Jeffrey Gold and his colleagues write that "acupuncture may serve to harmonize traditional Western medicine and Traditional Chinese medicine as a means of promoting preventive care and symptom management for children given the promising trends in the current acupuncture research, the relative willingness of families to engage in acupuncture and the low risk of deleterious side effects."

📝 New Words and Expressions

New Words and Expressions

cornerstone /ˈkɔːnəstəʊn/ n. a stone at the corner of the base of a building, often laid in a special ceremony 基石；奠基石

sterile /ˈsteraɪl/ adj. something that is sterile is completely clean and free from germs 无菌的

acupoint /ˈækjʊˌpɔɪnt/ n. any of the specific points on the body where a needle is inserted in acupuncture or pressure is applied in acupressure 穴位

elicit /ɪˈlɪsɪt/ v. call forth (emotions, feelings, and responses) 引起（反应）

meridian /məˈrɪdiən/ n. 1. one of the lines that is drawn from the North Pole to the South Pole on a map of the world 子午线；经线；2. pathways throughout human body 经脉；经络

vessel /ˈvesl/ n. a tube that carries blood through the body of a person or an animal, or liquid through the parts of a plant（人或动物的）血管；脉管；（植物的）导管

dysfunction /disˈfʌŋkʃn/ n. (medicine) any disturbance in the function of an organ or body part 功能紊乱；机能障碍

electrical grid a complex network that distributes electricity from power plants to end users 电力网

free up to make something available for use, or to release something that is not currently being used 释放

neurochemical /ˌnjuərəʊˈkemikəl/ *n.* any organic substance that occurs in neural activity 神经化学物质

endorphin /enˈdɔːfɪn/ *n.* (biology 生物) a hormone produced in the brain that reduces the feeling of pain 内啡肽(内分泌激素，有镇痛作用)

seek out to deliberately look for or try to find something or someone 挑选出；找出

menstrual /ˈmenstruəl/ *adj.* connected with the time when a woman menstruates each month 月经的

speed up to increase the pace or rate at which something happens (使)加速

subdue /səbˈdjuː/ *v.* to bring sb. /sth. under control, especially by using force 制服；征服；控制

modulate /ˈmɒdjuleɪt/ *v.* to affect sth. so that it becomes more regular, slower, etc. 调整；调节；控制

misfire /ˌmɪsˈfaɪə(r)/ *v.* (of a plan or joke) to fail to have the effect that you had intended 不奏效；不起作用

enkephalin /enˈkefəlin/ *n.* an endorphin having opiate qualities that occurs in the brain and spinal cord and elsewhere (生化) 脑啡肽

stave off to prevent something from happening or to delay its onset 避开；延缓

optimal /ˈɒptiməl/ *adj.* most desirable possible under a restriction expressed or implied 最佳的；最优化的

stagnation /stægˈneɪʃən/ *n.* a state of inactivity (in business or art etc.) inactivity of liquids; being stagnant; standing still; without current or circulation 停滞；停止

nitric oxide /ˈnaɪtrɪk ˈɒksaɪd/ *n.* a poisonous red-brown gas 一氧化氮

leukotrienes /ˌljuːkəʊˈtrɪənz/ *n.* a class of lipid compounds that play significant roles in inflammation and immune responses 白细胞三烯

anti-histamine /ˌæntiˈhɪstəˌmiːn/ *n.* antihistamine is a drug that is used to treat allergies 抗组胺剂

dilate /daɪˈleɪt/ *v.* to become or to make sth. larger, wider or more open 扩大；(使)膨胀；扩张

viscosity /vɪˈskɒsəti/ *n.* the quality of a fluid or semifluid that causes it to resist flowing and to move or spread slowly when subjected to stress 黏稠度

pathogenic /ˌpæθəˈdʒenɪk/ *adj.* causing disease; relating to pathogens 致病的；病原的；发病的

cholesterol /kəˈlestərɒl/ *n.* a type of fat that is present in the blood and in animal fats and oils. High levels of cholesterol in the blood increase the risk of heart disease 胆固醇

blood clot a gel-like mass of platelets and fibrin that forms when blood changes from a liquid to a solid state 血栓

regimen /ˈredʒɪmən/ *n.* a method of treatment, especially when used regularly and over a long period of time 治疗方案；生活方式

stringent /ˈstrɪndʒənt/ *adj.* (especially of financial measures) severe or harsh in its effects; rigorous 严格的；严厉的

portfolio /ˈpɔːtˈfəʊliəʊ/ *n.* the range of products or services offered by a particular company or organization(公司或机构提供的) 系列产品；系列服务；投资组合

fertilization /ˌfɜːrtɪlaɪˈzeɪʃən/ *n.* the process by which a female egg-cell is fertilized 受精

fertility /fəˈtɪlɪti/ *n.* the ability to produce offspring, especially in large numbers 生育能力；肥沃度

sterility /stəˈrɪlɪti/ *n.* the condition of being unable to reproduce, or the quality of being barren or infertile 不育；贫瘠

endocrinologist /ˌendəʊkrɪˈnɒlədʒɪst/ *n.* a scientist who specializes in endocrinology 内分泌学家

pediatric /ˌpiːdiˈætrɪk/ *adj.* relating to or concerned with the medical care of children 儿科的；小儿科的

intern /ɪnˈtɜːn/ *n.* a person who works for a company or organization as a trainee, typically for a fixed period after graduation 实习生；住院医生

affiliated /əˈfɪlieɪtɪd/ *adj.* connected or associated with something else, especially in a way that is formal or official 附属的；有关联的

serve to to be useful or beneficial for a specific purpose or function 有助于

deleterious /ˌdeləˈtiəriəs/ *adj.* harmful or damaging 有害的；有毒的

side effect an unintended and often undesirable secondary effect that occurs as a result of taking a medication, undergoing a medical procedure, or adopting a treatment 副作用

Notes

1. qi：In Traditional Chinese Medicine (TCM), the concept of qi or chi has two main branches. TCM believes that qi and blood are two basic substances in the human body, and occupy a very important position in human life activities. Qi can lead blood, qi can produce blood, qi can guide blood, and qi can absorb blood. Blood is the mother of qi, which can nourish qi and carry qi.

中医中，气的概念有两大分支。中医认为气与血是人体内的两大类基本物质，在人体生命活动中占有很重要的地位。气为血之帅，气能生血，气能行血，气能摄血。血为气之母，既能养气，也能载气。

2. NCCAM：The National Center for Complementary and Alternative Medicine (NCCAM) is one of the 27 institutes and centers that make up the National Institutes of Health (NIH) within the Department of Health and Hunan Services of the federal government of the United States. It investigates complementary and alternative medicine (CAM) healing practices in the context of rigorous scientific methodology, in training complementary and alternative medicine researchers, and in disseminating authoritative information to the public and professionals.

美国国家补充和替代医学中心是隶属于美国联邦政府卫生及公共服务部国立卫生研究院的27个研究中心之一，主要调查研究在严格的科学方法下的补充与替代治疗方法，提供补充与替代医学培训，并向大众及专业人员传播有关补充与替代医学的权威信息。

3. IVF：IVF (in vitro fertilization) is a type of fertility treatment where eggs are combined with sperm outside of your body in a lab. It's a method used by people who need help achieving pregnancy. IVF involves many complex steps and is an effective form of assisted reproductive technology (ART).

试管婴儿(体外受精)是一种生育治疗方法,在实验室中,卵子与精子在体外结合。这是需要人工受孕的人使用的方法。体外受精涉及许多复杂的步骤,是辅助生殖技术(ART)的有效形式。

4. Tao of Wellness：Tao of Wellness is a premiere Chinese medicine center in Southern California. Tao of Wellness and its predecessor clinic were established by Master Ni in 1976. All doctors and associates at Tao of Wellness treat various conditions, such as infertility, gynecological disorders, immunology, gastrointestinal, pain disorders, pain management and healthy ageing medicine.

该诊所是美国南加州的首个传统中医诊所,由倪大师于1976年创建。该诊所的医生能治疗包括不孕不育、妇科疾病、免疫力低下、肠胃疾病、疼痛症等疾病以及研制健康的抗衰老药物。

5. CHLA：Children's Hospital Los Angeles (CHLA) is a nonprofit institution that provides pediatric health care and helps the patients more than 528,000 times each year in a setting designed just for their needs. As the first and largest pediatric hospital in Southern California, CHLA relies on the generosity of philanthropists in the community to support compassionate patient care, leading-edge education of the caregivers of tomorrow and innovative research efforts that impact children at the hospital and around the world.

洛杉矶儿童医院是一家非营利性医院,专门提供儿科医疗保健并且每年就患者的需要给他们提供定制帮助多达52.8万次。作为美国南加州第一家而且最大的一家儿童医院,其经费主要来源于当地社区的慈善捐赠,并以此来资助医生义诊、给未来的护理人员提供前沿的教育知识以及提供对在院的和全球的病患儿童有帮助的创新性科研技术成果。

6. Yo San University of traditional Chinese Medicine：Yo San University, located in LA, is a non-profit organization dedicated to the education and inspiration of Traditional Chinese Medicine practitioners with an emphasis in the Taoist healing arts and collaborative care.

悠山中医药大学是一家坐落于洛杉矶的非营利性机构,致力于推动和鼓励中医药执业,强调道家的诊疗艺术和合作护理。

▣ After Reading Activities

Reading Comprehension

❤ I. Answer the following questions.

1. How does qi work to maintain health in the body?

2. Why is acupuncture an effective way to relieve pain?

3. What will happen when blood is blocked or nerves fail to communicate properly?

4. How do you understand the sentence "where there is stagnation there is disease, where there is disease there is stagnation".

5. According to Dr. Jefferey Gold and his colleagues, how does acupuncture work in the pediatrics?

❤ II. Work in groups to complete the following chart according to the structure of the text.

The introduction: (paras. 1-2)

    Acupuncture is part of a medical system called _____ that has been in continuous use for five thousand years and is the _____ of a civilization of nearly 1.4 billion people.

How does Acupuncture work: (para. 3)

    As long as qi flows freely throughout the _____, health is maintained, but once the flow of energy is blocked, the system is disrupted and _____ occur. So, acupuncture works to _____ and _____ normal function by stimulating certain points on the meridians in order to _____ the qi energy.

Six functions of Acupuncture: (paras. 4-15)

1. Calling the right _____ and _____;

2. Getting _____ to flow;

3. Acupuncture found beneficial for_____;

4. Acupuncture found to helpful for_____;

5. Acupuncture found to increase_____ ;

6. Pediatric acupuncture program helps children with_____ .

Words and Phrases

✔ I. Translate the following medical terms into Chinese or English.

1. elicit a healing response _____

2. pain relief _____

3. anti-inflammatory protein _____

4. pediatric acupuncture _____

5. 虚证 _____

6. 实证 _____

7. 月经痛 _____

8. 血块 _____

✔ II. Fill in the blanks with the words or phrases given below. Change the form if necessary.

fertility	modulate	stagnation	regimen	serve to

1. She is able to _____ and manage her emotional life in a dramatically better way.

2. The _____ of women who smoke is half that of nonsmoking women.

3. It's not high mountains and deep valleys that best _____ defend a country.

4. Where there is _____ there is disease.

5. Researchers have suggested that the _____ is easier than daily caloric restriction, but is it easy enough?

Sentence Translation

Translate the following sentences into Chinese or English.

1. Acupuncture may serve to harmonize traditional Western medicine and Traditional Chinese medicine as a means of promoting preventive care and symptom management for children

given the promising trends in the current acupuncture research, the relative willingness of families to engage in acupuncture and the low risk of deleterious side effects.

_____

_____

2. Health is preserved as long as this energy is allowed to freely move through the meridians.

_____

_____

3. Over 40% of individuals who had acupuncture during an IVF round were able to conceive, as opposed to 26% of pregnant patients who did not undergo the therapy.

_____

_____

4. 针刺疗法通过刺激经络上的穴位可以释放气，从而重新调和并恢复人体的正常机能。

_____

_____

5. 人体中的气通过经络运行体内。只要行气通畅，身体就会保持健康。但是一旦行气受阻，人体内阴阳平衡遭到破坏，疼痛和人体机能功能紊乱就会随之而来。

_____

_____

Text B

Pre-reading Questions:

1. What do you know about Traditional Chinese Medicine?

2. Which TCM treatments would you like to choose if you were sick? Give your reasons.

An Overview of Traditional Chinese Medicine (TCM)

Text B

What is Traditional Chinese Medicine?

1. The term "traditional Chinese medicine" refers to a catch-all term of medical procedures and methods that have evolved over hundreds or even thousands of years in China. Practitioners of TCM approach health from a holistic perspective. Rather than addressing individual symptoms, they consider the body as a whole using a holistic approach and seek to discover the disease's fundamental roots.

2. Qi is one of the central ideas in TCM. Qi is an essential energy that moves via channels known as meridians to circulate throughout the body. Qi flows freely in healthy persons, but obstructions in the flow or imbalances in its strength or weakness can lead to health issues. The goal of many TCM treatments is to get qi flowing again normally.

3. Doctors of TCM hold that the body's various organs and systems are interrelated and constitute an organic whole. You can characterize each component of this totality as either yang or yin. Unbalances in a person's yin and yang can occur if the blood is stagnant or if the flow of qi is hindered. Many TCM therapies center on restoring this equilibrium because imbalances like this are seen to be the root cause of health issues in Traditional Chinese Medicine.

4. Before choosing a course of treatment, Traditional Chinese Medicine (TCM) physicians frequently check their patients' tongues and take their pulses. Traditional Chinese Medicine (TCM) practitioners employ a range of diagnostic techniques, such as inquiry, inspection, palpation, olfaction (smelling) and auscultation (listening) for the final diagnosis.

TCM Treatments Commonly Used

Herbal medicines

5. Herbs are used in traditional Chinese medicine to treat the whole person and their symptoms. Herbs are prepared in capsule form, teas or extracts, and powders, in traditional or custom formulas. Herbal remedies are unlike pharmaceuticals used in Western medicine, which target specific disease symptoms. Many herbs may help with hard-to-diagnose or -treat syndromes, including allergies, infertility, and menopause.

Acupuncture

6. Acupuncture is when a practitioner stimulates specific points on the body by inserting thin needles through the skin. It is one of the most well-evidenced methods used in Traditional Chinese Medicine, although study results do vary. Clinical research reviews suggest acupuncture helps the body release natural painkillers and may be effective in helping reduce symptoms in patients with chronic (ongoing) pain.

Moxibustion

7. Moxibustion, which is frequently combined with acupuncture, is burning a herbal concoction on an acupuncture needle or directly on the body at key spots. It is believed that the heat produced by burning the herbs will help qi move throughout the meridians.

Massage

8. A unique kind of TCM therapy called tuina blends acupressure and massage methods. To aid enhance the flow of qi, practitioners apply firm, deep pressure to particular places along the meridians.

Cupping

9. In order to improve the flow of qi, cupping therapy involves applying rounded, inverted cups to the skin. Practitioners typically burn flammable material inside the cups before inserting them to produce a vacuum that makes the cups adhere firmly to the skin.

10. When removed, the cups leave circular dark purple bruises that can take up to three weeks to disappear. Cupping is used to treat headaches, nasal congestion, and various other types of ailments and pain.

Guasha

11. The practice of guasha entails pressing and rubbing the skin with a tool in an effort to

stimulate the body's flow of qi and stagnant blood. Guasha is frequently used to relieve tense muscles and joints.

12. Like cupping, this treatment leaves bruises on the skin which take some time to heal. For a fascinating exploration of East-West cultural misunderstandings with regard to guasha, check out the movie *The Guasha Treatment*.

Tai chi

13. Tai chi, two slow, meditative martial arts-inspired workouts, require practitioners to do a series of motions linked with regulated breathing exercises. These procedures are supposed to improve health and aid in qi balance in patients. Although they originated as martial arts, they have been incorporated into the TCM method set to support the balance of yin and yang and encourage appropriate qi flow.

Diet and nutrition

14. TCM practitioners believe certain foods are either "hot" or "cold" foods. Certain diseases are thought to result from an overabundance of either yang or yin in the body.

15. Dietary changes are able to address this excess. For instance, patients with too much yin may be advised to eat "hot" meals like mutton, while those with too much yang may be encouraged to eat "cold" foods like mung beans. TCM customs also advise people to modify their diets according to the seasons, consuming different foods in the summer and winter.

What is the Global Perception of Traditional Chinese Medicine?

16. In 1971, a piece by James Reston, a *New York Times* reporter who had appendicitis and had acupuncture treatment while traveling in China with Henry Kissinger, helped TCM become more well known in the United States. Since then, TCM has gained some traction in the United States and other Western nations as an alternative therapy.

17. In the early years of the People's Republic of China, the Chinese government sent TCM doctors to Africa as part of their foreign medical aid to the continent. More recently, China has actively promoted TCM internationally as the country works to expand its soft power abroad and secure a stake in the increasingly lucrative global TCM market.

18. China supports TCM tourism, which brings patients from all over the world to China, and offers government-sponsored training programs for international students interested in studying the practice. As part of the Belt and Road Initiative, it has also established TCM medical clinics in other cities throughout the world, such as Dubai and Barcelona, and it plans to open more. China donated medical professionals and supplies related to traditional medicine to nations impacted by the COVID-19 pandemic.

19. China successfully lobbied in 2019 for Traditional Chinese Medicine (TCM) to be listed in the International Statistical Classification of Diseases and Related Health Problems (ICD) of the World Health Organization. It is influential because it is a standard reference used by physicians, epidemiologists, health officials, insurance companies, and more than 100 other countries. The incorporation of TCM methods into this document is anticipated to hasten their global dissemination and ultimately facilitate that they become an integral part of the global health care system.

The Future of Traditional Chinese Medicine

20. Due to the recent addition of Traditional Chinese Medicine (TCM) to the World Health Organization's (WHO) important ICD document, TCM is anticipated to gain worldwide recognition. Numerous individuals, both domestically and abroad, find its holistic, reasonably peaceful, and affordable therapy methods appealing. TCM may be quite effective in treating a number of illnesses, particularly long-term issues like heart disease.

21. Short-term, widespread acceptance of many traditional Chinese remedies may be hampered by the absence of scientific proof of their efficacy. Standardizing TCM therapies and assessing their efficacy using contemporary scientific techniques require more effort. It might even become necessary in the end to develop new techniques that are better suited for assessing TCM treatments that originated outside of the Western medical paradigm.

22. It is more likely that ineffective TCM approaches will be discarded or modified as more research is done and data mounts, while more widely accepted TCM techniques will likely gain popularity in China and abroad.

✍ New Words and Expressions

catch-all term a term or word that can be used to represent many different things or concepts 万能术语

holistic /həʊˈlɪstɪk/ *adj.* relating to or involving holism; considering things as a whole, rather than separately 整体的；全息的

stagnant /ˈstægnənt/ *adj.* not flowing or changing; not developing or advancing 停滞的；不流动的

pulse /pʌls/ *n.* a regular beating of the heart that you can feel in your arteries as a series of beats 脉搏

palpation /pælˈpeɪʃn/ *n.* the act of examining part of the body by touching it gently with the hands 触诊

olfaction /ɒlˈfækʃn/ *n.* the act of using the sense of smell for diagnostic purposes 嗅觉；嗅诊

auscultation /ˌɔːskəlˈteɪʃn/ *n.* the act of listening to body sounds (as the heartbeat or breathing) for diagnostic purposes 听诊

diagnosis /ˌdaɪəgˈnəʊsɪs/ *n.* the art of identifying a disease from its signs and symptoms 诊断

capsule /ˈkæpsjuːl/ *n.* a small container made of gelatin, plastic, etc., that is filled with medicine 胶囊

formula /ˈfɔːmjələ/ *n.* a list of the things that sth. is made from, giving the amount of each substance to use 配方；处方；药方

pharmaceutical /ˌfɑːməˈsuːtɪkl/ *n.* a drug or medicine 药物

hard-to-diagnose /hɑːd tuː ˌdaɪəgˈnəʊs/ difficult to diagnose 难以诊断的

syndrome /ˈsɪndrəʊm/ *n.* a set of symptoms occurring together and characteristic of a particular disorder 综合征

menopause /ˈmenəpɔːz/ *n.* the period in a woman's life when menstruation stops permanently, typically occurring between the ages of 45 and 55 更年期

practitioner /præk'tɪʃənər/ n. a person who practices a particular profession or an occupation 从业者；执业者

painkiller /'peɪnkɪlər/ n. medication used to relieve pain 止痛药

moxibustion /mɒksɪ'bʌstʃən/ n. a traditional Chinese medical treatment in which a burning substance (such as moxa) is applied to or held close to the skin 艾灸

acupressure /'ækjupreʃər/ n. a form of therapy in which pressure is applied to specific parts of the body 穴位按压

cupping /'kʌpɪŋ/ n. a form of alternative therapy in which special cups are put on the skin to create a vacuum 拔罐

inverted /ɪn'vɜːrtɪd/ adj. turned upside down or inside out 倒转的；反转的

vacuum /'vækjuːm/ n. a space that is empty of all matter 真空

nasal congestion a condition in which the nose is blocked and cannot be easily cleared 鼻塞

ailment /'eɪlmənt/ n. an illness or disease, especially a minor one 疾病；小病

joint /dʒɔɪnt/ n. the place where two bones meet and move against each other, allowing movement of the body 关节

meditative /'medɪtətɪv/ adj. engaged in or characterized by meditation 冥想的

overabundance /'əʊvərə'bʌndəns/ n. an excessive amount or number; more than enough 过量；过剩

appendicitis /ə,pendə'saɪtɪs/ n. inflammation of the vermiform appendix, usually with infection and abscess formation 阑尾炎

alternative therapy a type of medical treatment that uses methods different from those of conventional Western medicine 替代疗法

continent /'kɒntɪnənt/ n. a very large land mass (especially considered as one of the seven divisions of the earth's surface) 大陆

stake /steɪk/ n. an important part or share in a business, plan, etc. that is important to you and that you want to be successful(在公司、计划等中的)重大利益；重大利害关系

lucrative /'luːkrətɪv/ adj. producing wealth; profitable 有利可图的

lobby /'lɒbi/ v. ~ (sb.) (for/against sth.) to try to influence a politician or the government and, for example, persuade them to support or oppose a change in the law 游说(从政者或政府)

influential /ˌɪnfluˈenʃl/ *adj.* having or exercising influence; having power to affect the outcome of events 有影响力的

integral /ˈɪntɪɡrəl/ *adj.* essential to a complete whole; forming an essential component of a system or structure 构成整体所必需的

discard /dɪsˈkɑːd/ *v.* to throw away as worthless or no longer useful or wanted 丢弃; 抛弃

Notes

1. *The Guasha Treatment*: a movie produced by Director Zheng Xiaolong, in the year 2001. The story is about misunderstanding between American and Oriental culture. After years of hard work, Xu Datong, a Chinese immigrant to the U.S., has finally achieved success as an outstanding video game designer. With his promising career and loving family, he feels he has become a true American. Datong's father comes over from China, and uses a traditional Chinese medical technique, called Guasha, to treat Datong's son, Dennis. Unexpectedly, an American doctor thinks the bruises on Dennis' back left by the Guasha treatment are signs of child abuse, and the finger is pointed at Datong. The Treatment is a moving portrayal of the enormous gulfs between cultures and their possible repercussions.

这是一部由郑晓龙导演在 2001 年执导的电影。故事讲述了美国与东方文化之间的误解。经过多年的努力,移民到美国的中国移民许大同终于成功成为了一名杰出的电子游戏设计师。他有着光明的职业生涯和充满爱的家庭,感觉自己已经成为了一位真正的美国人。大同的父亲从中国到美国,使用一种传统的中医技术——刮痧——来给大同的儿子丹尼斯治病。出乎意料的是,一位美国医生认为刮痧治疗后留在丹尼斯背上的瘀伤是虐待儿童的迹象,虐待的指责指向了大同。《刮痧》是一个感人的故事,描绘了文化之间巨大的鸿沟及其可能带来的后果。

2. Henry Kissinger（1923-2023）: the U.S. nation's 56th secretary of state, played a key role in influencing U.S. foreign policy on a global stage. Awarded the Nobel Peace Prize in 1973 for his part in trying to negotiate an end to the Vietnam War, he gained global fame for his strong, pragmatic influence in international diplomacy. Kissinger also engaged with China

in 1972, setting the stage for Nixon's pivotal visit to the communist nation to meet with Chairman Mao Zedong—the first time a sitting U.S. president had visited China's mainland and seen as a Cold War turning point.

亨利·基辛格(1923—2023)，美国第 56 任国务卿，他在影响美国在全球舞台上的外交政策方面发挥了关键作用。1973 年，他致力于通过谈判结束越南战争而被授予诺贝尔和平奖，他在国际外交上的强大而务实的影响力为他赢得了国际声誉。基辛格还在 1972 年与中国接触，为尼克松对中国的访问和会见毛泽东主席奠定了关键基础——这是美国总统首次访问中国大陆，并被视为冷战的转折点。

3. Belt and Road Initiative：The Belt and Road Initiative refers to the Silk Road Economic Belt and the 21st Century Maritime Silk Road proposed by Chinese President Xi Jinping in 2013. The initiative aims at promoting policy coordination, facilities connectivity, unimpeded trade, financial integration and people-to-people bond in the international community. The concept of the Belt and Road Initiative is inspired by the ancient Silk Road that witnessed hundreds of years of booming trade and cultural exchange on the Eurasian continent. The newly launched Belt and Road intends to bring countries in the world closer than ever.

"一带一路"倡议是指 2013 年习近平主席提出的丝绸之路经济带和 21 世纪海上丝绸之路。"一带一路"旨在促进国际社会政策沟通、设施联通、贸易畅通、资金融通、民心相通。"一带一路"倡议的灵感来源于古老的丝绸之路，这条丝绸之路见证了欧亚大陆数百年的贸易和文化交流。新启动的"一带一路"旨在将世界各国比以往任何时候都更紧密地联系在一起。

4. International Statistical Classification of Diseases and Related Health Problems (ICD)：ICD serves a broad range of uses globally and provides critical knowledge on the extent, causes and consequences of human disease and death worldwide via data that is reported and coded with the ICD. Clinical terms coded with ICD are the main basis for health recording and statistics on disease in primary, secondary and tertiary care, as well as on cause of death certificates.

《国际疾病分类》在全球范围内获得广泛使用，并通过所报告和编码的数据提供关于全球人类疾病和死亡的程度、原因和后果的关键知识。以《国际疾病分类》编码的临床术语是初级、二级和三级保健中健康记录和疾病统计以及死亡原因证明的主要依据。

📝 After Reading Activities

Reading Comprehension

Decide whether the following statements are true (T) or false (F) according to the text.

_____ 1. TCM applies a holistic approach. Instead of treating specific symptoms of a disease in isolation, they look at the body as a whole and work to identify the underlying causes of the disease.

_____ 2. If the flow of qi is blocked or the blood is stagnant, imbalances in a person's yin and yang can result. According to TCM, these imbalances can lead to health problems, so many TCM therapies focus on restoring this balance.

_____ 3. Cupping therapy involves placing inverted rounded cups onto the skin to inhibit the flow of qi and blood.

_____ 4. In the short term, the lack of scientific evidence to prove the efficacy of many traditional Chinese therapies may hinder their popularity. More work is needed to standardize TCM treatments.

_____ 5. TCM has enjoyed some popularity as a standard therapy in the U.S. and other Western countries.

Words and Phrases

Match each English phrase in Column A with its Chinese version in Column B.

Column A	Column B
1. holistic approach	A. 鼻塞
2. alternative therapy	B. 瘀血
3. herbal remedies	C. 整体综合方法
4. traditional formulas	D. 草药疗法
5. nasal congestion	E. 把脉
6. stagnant blood	F. 传统方剂
7. soft power	G. 替代疗法
8. take patients' pulse	H. 软实力

Translation

中医认为，人体内所有不同的器官和系统形成一个相互联系的有机整体。这个整体的每一部分都可以被描述为阴或阳。如果气血流动受阻，就会导致人体阴阳失衡。根据中医的说法，这些不平衡会导致健康问题，所以许多中医疗法都专注于恢复这种平衡。在诊断时，中医医生使用各种方法，包括询问、检查、触诊、嗅觉（闻）和听诊（听）。在决定疗程之前，中医医生通常会给病人把脉和检查他们的舌头。

_____

_____

_____

_____

Critical Thinking

TCM may have great potential for treating certain ailments, especially chronic conditions like heart disease, and is now gaining popularity in many countries globally. While others think traditional Chinese medicine should not be used in replacement of Western medicine or to delay the possibility of treatment for serious disorders, infections, or the like. As a student of medicine, what's your opinion on TCM and western medicine, and on their collaboration in the future?

Part III　Apply Medical English

✅ A. Situational Dialogues in Different Clinical Departments

Traditional Chinese Medicine（中医科）

Headaches and Insomnia（头痛和失眠）

Dialogue

Doctor：Good morning, how can I assist you today?

Patient：Hello, doctor. I've been struggling with frequent headaches and insomnia lately, and I was hoping to explore acupuncture as a possible treatment.

Doctor：I'm sorry to hear that you're experiencing these symptoms. Before we proceed, could you please tell me more about your headaches and sleep patterns? How long have you been dealing with these issues?

Patient：The headaches have been bothering me for a few months now. They usually start as a dull ache and then escalate into a throbbing pain, especially around my temples. As for my sleep, I've been having trouble falling asleep and staying asleep throughout the night for about the same amount of time.

Doctor：I see. Have you noticed any particular triggers for your headaches or any patterns in your sleep disturbances?

Patient：Well, I haven't been able to pinpoint any specific triggers for the headaches, but they tend to worsen when I'm stressed or fatigued. As for my sleep, I've noticed that I often wake up feeling restless and unable to relax.

Doctor：Thank you for sharing that information. Now, I'd like to take a moment to observe your overall appearance and demeanor. Could you please roll up your sleeves so I can take a look at your wrists?

Patient：Of course, doctor.

[*The doctor observes the patient's complexion, posture, and general appearance, as well as the condition of the patient's tongue.*]

Doctor: Based on what I've observed, you appear to have a pale complexion, which is often associated with deficient energy or blood circulation. Your tongue also shows signs of slight coating and swelling, indicating potential internal imbalances.

Patient: That's interesting. What does that mean for my treatment?

Doctor: These observations, along with the information you've provided about your symptoms, suggest that there may be underlying imbalances in your body's energy flow, which is commonly addressed through acupuncture in Traditional Chinese Medicine (TCM). Now, if you don't mind, I'd like to feel your pulse to further assess your condition.

[*The doctor takes the patient's pulse at various points on the wrist and notes the strength, rhythm, and quality of the pulse.*]

Doctor: Your pulse feels slightly weak and irregular, particularly in the positions corresponding to the heart and kidney meridians. This further supports the possibility of energy imbalances contributing to your headaches and sleep disturbances.

Patient: I see. So, how can acupuncture help rebalance my energy and alleviate my symptoms?

Doctor: Acupuncture works by stimulating specific points along the body's meridian pathways to regulate the flow of qi and blood, thereby addressing imbalances and promoting healing. By targeting points associated with the heart, kidneys, and other relevant meridians, we can help alleviate your headaches, improve your sleep quality, and restore overall well-being.

Patient: That sounds promising. I'm willing to give it a try. When can we schedule my first acupuncture session?

Doctor: Wonderful! Let's go ahead and set up your initial appointment. In the meantime, I'll also provide you with some dietary and lifestyle recommendations to support your treatment and optimize your health outcomes.

Patient: Thank you so much, doctor. I appreciate your thorough assessment and guidance.

📇 Words and Phrases

dull ache /dʌl eɪk/ *n.* 隐痛，通常被描述为一种钝痛或隐隐作痛的感觉

escalate /ˈeskəleɪt/ *v.* 加剧；恶化

throbbing pain /ˈθrɒbɪŋ peɪn/ *n.* 通常伴随着心跳或脉搏的悸动感

temples /ˈtemplz/ *n.* 太阳穴

sleep disturbances /sliːp dɪsˈtɜːbənsɪz/ 睡眠障碍

pinpoint /ˈpɪnpɔɪnt/ *v.* 明确指出；确定(位置或时间)

fatigued /fəˈtiːgd/ *adj.* 身心交瘁；精疲力竭

demeanor /dɪˈmiːnə/ *n.* 举止

pale complexion /peɪl kəmˈplekʃn/ 苍白的脸色

deficient energy /dɪˈfɪʃnt ˈenədʒi/ 气虚

slight coating and swelling /slaɪt ˈkəʊtɪŋ ənd ˈswelɪŋ/ 舌苔偏厚并肿胀

underlying imbalances /ˌʌndəˈlaɪɪŋ ɪmˈbælənsɪz/ 潜在的失衡

heart and kidney meridians /hɑːt ənd ˈkɪdni məˈrɪdɪənz/ 心经和肾经

alleviate /əˈliːvieɪt/ *v.* 减轻；缓和；缓解

📇 Notes

In Traditional Chinese Medicine（TCM），diagnosis typically involves a holistic approach that considers various aspects of a patient's health and well-being. Here are the usual procedures a TCM doctor might follow：

Initial Consultation

The doctor begins by conducting a thorough interview with the patient to gather information about their medical history, current symptoms, lifestyle, diet, emotions, and any other relevant factors.

Four Examinations（Si Zhen）

Inspection：The doctor observes and inspects the patient's appearance, including complexion, posture, movements, facial expressions, and any visible signs such as swelling, discoloration, or skin conditions. They may also examine the patient's tongue for color, coating, moisture, and any unusual features, as the tongue is believed to reflect the condition of internal organs.

Listening and Smelling: The doctor pays attention to the patient's voice, breathing, cough, and any odors that may be indicative of an underlying condition. Changes in voice tone or breathing patterns can provide valuable clues about the state of the patient's organs and energy flow.

Inquiry: The doctor asks detailed questions about the patient's symptoms, medical history, lifestyle habits, emotional state, and other relevant factors.

Palpation: The doctor feels the patient's pulse at various positions on the wrist to assess the quality, rhythm, strength, and other characteristics of the pulse.

Pattern Identification (Zhen Duan)

Based on the information gathered from the four examinations, the doctor analyzes the patient's symptoms, signs, and overall health condition to identify specific patterns of disharmony or imbalance. These patterns are classified according to TCM principles, such as excess or deficiency, heat or cold, and the involvement of specific organs or meridians.

Diagnosis and Treatment Plan

Finally, the doctor formulates a diagnosis based on the identified patterns of disharmony and develops a personalized treatment plan tailored to address the root causes of the patient's symptoms.

在中医中，诊断通常采用整体观，考虑患者健康和幸福的各个方面。以下是中医师可能遵循的常规程序：

初步咨询：

医生首先通过与患者进行全面的面诊来收集关于其病史、当前症状、生活方式、饮食、情绪和任何其他相关因素的信息。

四诊：

望诊：医生观察患者的外观，包括面色、姿势、动作、面部表情以及任何可见的迹象，如肿胀、变色或皮肤状况。他们还可以检查患者的舌头，观察颜色、舌苔、湿润度和任何异常特征，因为舌头被认为能够反映内脏的状况。

闻诊：医生注意患者的声音、呼吸、咳嗽以及可能表明患者内部状况的任何气味。声音音调或呼吸模式的变化可以提供关于患者器官和气血流动状态的有价值的线索。

问诊：医生详细询问患者的症状、病史、生活方式习惯、情绪状态和其他相关因素。

切诊：医生在感知患者腕部脉搏的各个位置时，评估脉搏的充盈度、节律、强度和其他特征。

辨证：

根据四诊收集的信息，医生分析患者的症状、体征和整体健康状况，识别特定的不和谐或失衡模式。这些模式根据中医原则进行分类，例如过度或不足、热或寒，以及特定器官或经络的参与情况。

诊断和治疗计划：

最后，医生根据识别出的不和谐模式制定诊断方案，并制定有针对性的治疗计划，旨在找出引发患者症状的根本原因，提出解决方案。

▣ Practical Activity

Work with your partner to create and perform a doctor-patient dialogue related to Traditional Chinese Medicine treatment.

✔ B. Practical Unit Project

Group Task：Please work in groups and present one of TCM treatments bilingually to our class using slides.

Guidance for Production

Guidelines for Structuring a Presentation：

1. Greet the audience and introduce yourself

Before you start delivering your talk, introduce yourself to the audience and clarify who you are and your relevant expertise. This does not need to be long or incredibly detailed, but will help build an immediate relationship between you and the audience.

2. Introduction

In the introduction, you need to explain the subject and purpose of your presentation whilst gaining the audience's interest and confidence. Keep in mind that the main aim of the introduction is to grab the audience's attention and connect with them.

3. The main body of your talk

The main body of your talk needs to meet the promises you made in the introduction. You can choose one TCM treatment to present its origin, history, function, feature, modern development, or future. Main points should be addressed one by one with supporting evidences and examples.

4. Conclusion

Be sure to summarize your main points and their implications. This clarifies the overall purpose of your talk and reinforces your reason for being there.

5. Thank the audience and invite questions

Conclude your talk by thanking the audience for their time and invite them to ask any questions they may have. Q and A is acceptable.

As for the slides, they are a useful tool for most presentations: they can greatly assist in the delivery of your message and help the audience follow along with what you are saying. Key slides include:

- An intro slide outlining your ideas
- A summary slide with core points to remember
- High quality image slides to supplement what you are saying

Golden Rules to Follow When Using Slides in a Presentation:

1. Don't over fill them: your slides are there to assist your speech, rather than be the focal point. They should have as little information as possible, to avoid distracting people from your talk.

2. A picture says a thousand words: instead of filling a slide with text, focus on one or two images or diagrams to help support and explain the point you are discussing at that time.

3. Make them readable: depending on the size of your audience, some may not be able to see small text or images, so make everything large enough to fill the space.

4. Don't rush through slides: give the audience enough time to digest each slide.

Part IV   Self-Assessment

Use the following self-assessment checklist to check what you have learned in this unit.

I understand the basic concept of TCM.	☐
I can identify and use the words, phrases and sentence patterns related to the topic.	☐
I can do the translation and make a presentation by using the terminologies and medical information of TCM.	☐
I can spread Chinese TCM to the world and make the whole world know more about TCM.	☐

Unit 5
Psychological Treatment

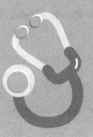

Psychological treatment is sometimes called psychotherapy or talking therapy. It involves talking about one's thoughts with a professional to better understand one's own thinking and behaviour, understand and resolve one's problems, recognize symptoms of mental illness in oneself, reduce symptoms, change behaviour and improve quality of life. Evidence shows that psychological treatments work well for emotional, mental and behavioral issues. Psychological treatments are useful for people of all ages,

Lead in

127

including children. They can help people from different cultural, social and language backgrounds. Psychiatrists can provide psychological treatments to people with mental illness. There are different types of psychological treatments designed to help with different issues.

This unit is mainly to achieve the following objectives:

1) Understand the basic concept of psychological treatment;

2) Identify words, phrases and sentence patterns related to the topic;

3) Make a conversation by using the terminologies and medical information in this unit;

4) Learn to embrace future life with a positive attitude.

Part I   View the Medical World

Watch a video about clinical depression and choose the right answer.①

1. Which one is the symptom of depression?

    A. Feeling excited.   B. Sleeping regularly.

    C. Changes in appetite.   D. Extensive socializing.

2. Depression has physical manifestations that can be seen with _____.

    A. X-ray vision   B. laser

    C. microscope   D. endoscope

3. Which of the following does NOT change during depression?

    A. Neurotransmitter.   B. Frontal lobe.

    C. Hippocampal volume.   D. Eyesight.

4. According to the video, depression symptoms are _____.

    A. predictable   B. intangible

    C. acceptable   D. curable

5. How long does it take an average person suffering with a mental illness to ask for help?

    A. About 10 years.   B. Over a decade.

    C. Nearly 10 years.   D. About a decade.

Words and Phrases

disorder /dɪsˈɔːdə(r)/ *n.* 失调；紊乱；不适；疾病

linger /ˈlɪŋɡə(r)/ *v.* 继续存留；缓慢消失

consecutive /kənˈsekjətɪv/ *adj.* 连续不断的

manifestation /ˌmænɪfeˈsteɪʃn/ *n.* 临床表现

---

① 视频详见网站：https://pan-yz. cldisk. com/external/m/file/1055138594360090624。

frontal lobe /ˈfrʌntlˈləʊb/ n. 额叶

hippocampal volume /ˌhɪpəˈkæmpəl ˈvɒljuːm/ 海马体积

norepinephrine /ˌnɔːrepɪˈnefrɪn/ n. 降肾上腺素；去甲肾上腺素

dopamine /ˈdəʊpəmiːn/ n. 多巴胺

REM（rapid eye movement）n.（夜间做梦时）眼部急速活动；快速眼动

cortisol /ˈkɔːtɪsɒl/ n. 皮质醇

thyroid hormone /ˈθaɪrɔɪd ˈhɔːməʊn/ n. 甲状腺激素

intangible /ɪnˈtændʒəbl/ adj. 难以形容（或理解）的；不易度量的

Part II   Read to Explore Medical Knowledge

Text A

Pre-reading Questions:

1. Do you know any effective ways to relief the stress that people have to deal with in their lives?

2. How can college students find help while facing psychological problems?

Medications to Psychotherapy: There's Often a Gray Area in Depression Treatment

Text A

1. Approximately 16 million Americans are afflicted by depression each year; many of them seek help from their physicians in desperation, embarking on a sometimes difficult process of figuring out what are their next steps. The process may entail completing questionnaires that include screening questions regarding symptoms such as changes in mood and sleep disturbances. Physicians may request patients to disclose personal information on topics such as marital disputes and suicidal tendencies. Certain individuals may be directed to mental health experts for additional assessment.

2. Patients often are asked after a depression diagnosis: "Are you interested in therapy, medications or both?"

3. In my experience as a resident physician in psychiatry, many patients grapple with this issue, and the response I hear most often is "I'm not sure." In the midst of a depressive episode, it can be quite difficult to decide between various forms of medical treatment. And we doctors aren't always sure of the best course of action for each given patient despite the fact that patients depend on us for guidance.

4. Although cognitive behavioral therapy (CBT) and other evidence-based therapies have

recently gained prominence in the area of psychotherapy, the public often associates it with Freud and couches. Cognitive behavioral therapy teaches patients how to change negative patterns of thinking, feeling, and behaving that could exacerbate their depression.

5. The mechanisms by which various psychotherapies alleviate depression have several postulated causes. Researchers are utilizing neuroimaging to examine the effects of potential therapies for depression, such as providing patients with social support and coping skills.

6. It is believed that antidepressant medicines alter brain chemical signaling pathways. For instance, selective serotonin reuptake inhibitors are a family of medications that aim to modify the levels of the neurotransmitter serotonin in the brain. We still don't fully understand how these antidepressants ease depressed symptoms, and although they may be helpful for treating depression in certain individuals, our understanding of the neurochemistry of depression is still lacking.

7. Several studies conducted recently highlight the ambiguity associated with these treatment choices. Researchers have extensively investigated the comparative efficacy of psychotherapies and antidepressants, often with little discernible distinction. A study conducted in 2012 analyzed data from over 100 previous trials involving more than 10,000 patients. The study found that both psychotherapies and antidepressants were more effective than a placebo in reducing depressive symptoms in blinded trials. However, there was no significant difference in effectiveness between these two treatments. Moreover, both psychotherapies and antidepressants have shown no superior efficacy compared to other treatments, such as exercise, when considering the overall outcomes.

8. Research presented at the 2014 European Congress of Psychiatry indicated that cognitive behavioral therapy was equally, if not more, effective than pharmaceuticals for the immediate treatment of depression. A comprehensive analysis conducted in 2015, which analyzed randomized trials, reached the same conclusion that antidepressants were not superior to cognitive behavioral therapy in controlling depression, as measured by several criteria. A recent meta-analysis examining several research discovered that psychotherapies and pharmaceuticals were very similar in their ability to enhance the quality of life and functioning of individuals with depression.

9. Could the combination of psychotherapy and medicine be even more effective in treating depression?

10. This question is valid and frequently raised by patients. However, the efficacy of

combining these therapies is controversial in medical circles. Various studies have yielded conflicting findings on this matter. Consequently, a significant number of patients continue to undergo any one of the treatments initially.

11. The American College of Physicians issued recommendations about the use of antidepressants in 2016 as opposed to non-pharmacologic treatments for depression. The committee's conclusion was that cognitive behavioral therapy and newer-generation antidepressants are "similarly effective treatments" for individuals with serious depression, based on a review of decades of research. The recommendations advise practitioners to choose either cognitive behavioral therapy or second-generation antidepressants as the preferred treatment options for individuals with depression.

12. The authors of these guidelines also highlight a crucial aspect: Physicians frequently prioritize the use of antidepressants as the initial treatment for patients with depression, despite data indicating that other treatments are as effective. The treatments may also induce side effects such as nausea and vomiting, as well as potentially hazardous combinations with other medications.

13. More than 250 million prescriptions for antidepressants are filled every year in the United States, making them one of the most prescribed forms of drugs. According to a 2015 *JAMA* research, the percentage of persons in the U.S. who used antidepressants in 2012 nearly doubled from 1999 to 2012.

14. Is the overprescribing of antidepressants a result of this?

15. The answer varies depending on the interpretation of the question. The utilization of antidepressants has significantly increased in recent years, while the utilization of psychotherapy seems to be steady or decreasing. This trend may indicate a growing dependence on medication, although both therapies are generally equally effective in controlling depression.

16. Medication for depression may be preferred by some people. Psychotherapies, such as cognitive behavioral therapy or psychodynamic therapy (a form of talk therapy that investigates the interplay between unconscious emotions and distressing symptoms), can span months and include several hour-long sessions, which is too much for many individuals. Some people might not be able to afford the treatment they need because they do not have access to mental health professionals. On the other hand, some people might

prefer to take medication at home rather than disclose personal information in a medical setting.

17. One possible contributing reason is the design of our health care system. Physicians may be more inclined to prescribe drugs instead of psychotherapies if they receive higher insurance reimbursements for pharmaceuticals. The crunched time and administrative demands of modern medical practice sometimes result in rushed patient appointments that are more conducive to efficiency and medication than to meaningful discussions.

18. Patients should know that they have alternatives to medicine and therapy when it comes to treatment choices. Exercise has shown promise in a number of trials for the treatment of mild to severe depression. Methods that employ short electric currents to affect brain function, such as transcranial magnetic stimulation and electroconvulsive therapy, can be lifesaving for individuals with more severe depression.

19. When treating depression, clinicians should talk with patients about "treatment effects, adverse effect profiles, cost, accessibility, and preferences," as advised by the ACP recommendations. However, it may sometimes be challenging, if not impossible, to do that duty in a full and comprehensive way in the current hectic medical environment.

20. Brain imaging and genetic testing are among the techniques that researchers are developing to aid in this decision-making process. People with mental health issues have long wished for more tailored treatments.

21. Although these technologies have demonstrated potential, they are still a long way from being widely adopted in clinical settings. Furthermore, the inclusion of additional examinations during doctors' visits may overlook the fundamental problem in the treatment of depression: Do we allocate sufficient time to engage in meaningful conversations with our patients on their available choices?

New Words and Expressions

New Words and
Expressions

psychotherapy /ˌsaɪkəʊˈθerəpi/ n. the treatment of mental illness by discussing sb.'s problems with them rather than by giving them drugs 心理治疗；精神治疗

afflict /əˈflɪkt/ v. to affect sb./sth. in an unpleasant or harmful way 折磨；使痛苦

embark on to start or begin a particular course of action, especially one that is difficult, complex, or adventurous 从事；着手

entail /ɪnˈteɪl/ v. to involve sth. that cannot be avoided 牵涉；需要；使必要

suicidal /ˌsuːɪˈsaɪdl/ adj. people who are suicidal feel that they want to kill themselves 想自杀的；有自杀倾向的

resident physician a medical doctor who has completed their undergraduate medical education and is training to become a specialist in a particular field of medicine 住院医师

psychiatry /saɪˈkaɪətri/ n. the study and treatment of mental illness 精神病学；精神病治疗

grapple with to struggle or wrestle with a problem, issue, or situation 努力克服

cognitive /ˈkɒgnətɪv/ adj. connected with mental processes of understanding 认知的；感知的；认识的

evidence-based /ˈevɪdənsbeɪst/ adj. based on evidence 基于证据的；循证的

alleviate /əˈliːvieɪt/ v. to make sth. less severe 减轻；缓和；缓解

neuroimaging /njʊərɔɪˈmædʒɪŋ/ n. the process of producing images of the structure or activity of the brain or other part of the nervous system by techniques such as magnetic resonance imaging or computerized tomography 神经影像

antidepressant /ˌæntidɪˈpresnt/ n. a drug used to treat depression 抗抑郁药

signaling /ˈsɪgnəlɪŋ/ n. any nonverbal action or gesture that encodes a message 打信号；发信号

serotonin /ˌserəˈtəʊnɪn/ n. a chemical in the brain that affects how messages are sent from the brain to the body, and also affects how a person feels 血清素；五羟色胺(神经递质，亦影响情绪等)

reuptake /riːˈʌpteɪk/ n. a process of using up or consuming again (神经细胞对化学物质的)再吸收；再摄取

inhibitor /ɪnˈhɪbɪtə(r)/ n. a substance which delays or prevents a chemical reaction 抑制剂；阻聚剂

neurotransmitter /ˈnjʊərəʊtrænzmɪtə(r)/ n. a chemical that carries messages from nerve cells to other nerve cells or muscles 神经递质(在神经细胞间或向肌肉传递信息)

neurochemistry /njʊərəˈkemɪstrɪ/ n. the branch of biochemistry concerned with the processes occurring in nerve tissue and the nervous system 神经化学

highlight /ˈhaɪlaɪt/ v. to emphasize sth., especially so that people give it more attention 突出；强调

placebo /pləˈsiːbəʊ/ n. a substance that has no physical effects, given to patients who do not need medicine but think that they do（给无实际治疗需要者的）安慰剂

blinded trial a type of research study in which the participants and the researchers are unaware of which group is receiving the experimental treatment and which is receiving the control treatment 盲法试验

overall /ˌəʊvərˈɔːl/ adv. generally; when you consider everything 一般来说；大致上；总体上

randomized trial a type of experimental study design in which participants are randomly assigned to one of two or more groups：an intervention group, which receives the treatment being studied, and a control group, which receives either a placebo, no treatment, or a different standard treatment 随机试验

valid /ˈvælɪd/ adj. based on what is logical or true 符合逻辑的；合理的；有根据的；确凿的

efficacy /ˈefɪkəsi/ n. the ability of sth., especially a drug or a medical treatment, to produce the results that are wanted（尤指药物或治疗方法的）功效；效验；效力

controversial /ˌkɒntrəˈvɜːʃl/ adj. causing a lot of angry public discussion and disagreement 引起争论的；有争议的

medical circle a group of medical professionals who share a common interest or focus in a specific area of medicine 医学界

as opposed to used to indicate a contrast or difference between two things 而不是

non-pharmacologic /nʌnˌfɑːməkəˈlɒdʒɪk/ adj. referring to therapy that does not involve drugs 非药物的

nausea /ˈnɔːziə/ n. the feeling that you have when you want to vomit, for example because you are ill/sick or are disgusted by sth. 恶心；作呕；反胃

vomiting /ˈvɒmɪtɪŋ/ n. to bring food from the stomach back out through the mouth 呕吐

overprescribe /ˈəʊvəprɪˈskraɪb/ v. prescribe (a drug or treatment) in greater amounts or on more occasions than necessary 处方过量；开(药)过量

interpretation /ɪnˌtɜːprɪˈteɪʃn/ n. the particular way in which sth. is understood or explained 理解；解释；说明

psychodynamic /ˌsaɪkəʊdaɪˈnæmɪk/ *adj.* of or relating to the interrelation of the unconscious and conscious mental and emotional forces that determine personality and motivation 心理动力的；神经动力的

interplay /ˈɪntəpleɪ/ *n.* the way in which two or more things or people affect each other 相互影响(或作用)

distressing /dɪˈstresɪŋ/ *adj.* making you feel extremely upset, especially because of sb.'s suffering 使人痛苦的；令人苦恼的

span /spæn/ *v.* to last all through a period of time or to cover the whole of it 持续；贯穿

reimbursement /ˌriːɪmˈbɜːsmənt/ *n.* to pay back money to sb. which they have spent or lost 偿还；补偿

crunched /krʌntʃt/ *adj.* not having enough of sth.；lacking sth. 不足；短缺

medical practice the professional activities of diagnosing, treating, and preventing diseases and other medical conditions 医疗实践；医务工作

conducive /kənˈdjuːsɪv/ *adj.* making it easy, possible or likely for sth. to happen 使容易(或有可能)发生的

promise /ˈprɒmɪs/ *n.* a sign that sb./sth. will be successful 获得成功的迹象

electric current the flow of electric charge in a conductor such as a metal wire 电流

transcranial /trænskˈræniəl/ *adj.* passing or performed through the skull 经颅的

magnetic /mæɡˈnetɪk/ *adj.* connected with or produced by magnetism 磁的；磁性的

electroconvulsive /ɪˌlektrəʊkənˈvʌlsɪv/ *adj.* of, relating to, or involving convulsive response to electroshock 电惊厥的；电休克的

profile /ˈprəʊfaɪl/ *n.* a description of sb./sth. that gives useful information 概述；简介

accessibility /əkˌsesəˈbɪlətɪ/ *n.* the quality of being able to be reached or entered 可达(及)性；可(易)接近性

📇 Notes

1. cognitive behavioral therapy: Cognitive behavioral therapy (CBT) is a common type of talk therapy. The patient works with a mental health counselor in a structured way, attending a limited number of sessions. CBT helps the patient become aware of inaccurate or negative

thinking so the patient can view challenging situations more clearly and respond to them in a more effective way.

认知行为疗法(CBT)是一种常见的谈话疗法。患者以结构化的方式与心理健康顾问一起参加一定数量的谈话。认知行为疗法可以帮助患者意识到不准确或消极的想法，这样患者就可以更清楚地看待具有挑战性的情况，并以更有效的方式应对。

2. selective serotonin reuptake inhibitors：Selective serotonin reuptake inhibitors (SSRIs) are a group of prescription medications prescribed to treat symptoms of depression, anxiety, and other mental health conditions. SSRIs treat depression by increasing levels of serotonin in the brain. Serotonin is one of the chemical messengers (neurotransmitters) that carry signals between brain nerve cells (neurons). SSRIs block the reabsorption (reuptake) of serotonin into neurons. This makes more serotonin available to improve transmission of messages between neurons. SSRIs are called selective because they mainly affect serotonin, not other neurotransmitters.

选择性血清素再摄取抑制剂(SSRIs)是一组处方药，用于治疗抑郁、焦虑和其他心理健康状况的症状。SSRIs通过提高大脑中血清素的水平来治疗抑郁症。血清素是在脑神经细胞(神经元)之间传递信号的化学信使(神经递质)之一。SSRIs阻断血清素向神经元的再吸收(再摄取)。这使得更多的血清素可以用来改善神经元之间的信息传递。SSRIs之所以被称为选择性，是因为它们主要影响血清素，而不是其他神经递质。

3. European Congress of Psychiatry：欧洲心理学大会

4. American College of Physicians：美国医师协会

5. JAMA：The Journal of the American Medical Association《美国医学会杂志》

6. Transcranial Magnetic Stimulation：Transcranial magnetic stimulation (TMS) is a procedure that uses magnetic fields to stimulate nerve cells in the brain to improve symptoms of major depression. During a TMS procedure, an electromagnetic coil is placed against the scalp of the head. This coil delivers magnetic pulses that stimulate nerve cells in the region of the brain involved in mood control and depression. It activates regions of the brain that have decreased activity during depression.

经颅磁刺激技术(TMS)是一种利用磁场刺激大脑中神经细胞以改善严重抑郁症症状的方法。在治疗过程中，一个电磁线圈被放在患者的头部。这个线圈提供磁脉冲，刺激大脑中与情绪控制和抑郁有关的区域的神经细胞。这可以激活大脑中在抑郁症期间活动减少的区域。

7. electroconvulsive therapy：Electroconvulsive therapy（ECT）, formerly known as electroshock therapy, is a procedure, done under general anesthesia, in which small electric currents are passed through the brain, intentionally triggering a brief seizure. ECT causes changes in brain chemistry that can quickly reverse symptoms of certain mental health conditions.

电惊厥疗法，曾被称为"电休克疗法"，是一种在全身麻醉下进行的手术。在这种手术中，小电流通过大脑，有意引发患者短暂的意识丧失。ECT 引起大脑化学物质的变化，可以迅速逆转某些心理健康状况的症状。

After Reading Activities

Reading Comprehension

I. Answer the following questions.

1. What are the treatments for depression mentioned in the passage?

2. Which treatment is more effective in treating depression, psychotherapies or antidepressants?

3. Why do some patients prefer to take antidepressants even though evidence suggests psychotherapies are just as effective?

4. What are the other treatment options in addition to psychotherapy and medication, according to the passage?

5. According to the recommendation from the ACP guidelines, what factors should clinicians talk with patients while treating depression?

II. Work in groups to complete the following chart according to the structure of the text.

The problem both patients and doctors facing：(paras. 1-3)

Depression afflicts an estimated _____ every year, many of whom go to their doctors in despair, _____ an often stressful process about what to do next. However, it is an uneasy task for both doctors and patients to decide between _____.

Unit 5 Psychological Treatment

The effectiveness of treatments for depression: (paras. 4-11)

Researchers have dedicated considerable effort to studying the relative effectiveness between ＿＿＿＿＿＿＿＿＿ and ＿＿＿＿＿＿＿＿＿, frequently without finding discernible distinction. But ＿＿＿＿＿＿＿ is controversial in medical circles. A committee concluded that CBT and newer-generation antidepressants are ＿＿＿＿＿＿＿＿＿ for individuals with serious depression.

Doctors' and patients' choice for treating depression and the reasons behind: (paras. 12-17)

Physicians frequently prioritize the use of ＿＿＿＿＿＿ when treating patients with depression, despite data indicating that ＿＿＿＿＿＿＿＿＿ are as effective.

＿＿＿＿＿＿＿＿ has significantly increased in recent years, while ＿＿＿＿＿＿＿＿ appears to be stable or declining. Psychotherapies can span months and include several hour-long sessions, which is ＿＿＿＿＿＿＿＿＿. Others might not be able to afford the treatment and they might not have access to ＿＿＿＿＿＿＿＿＿ who can provide appropriate therapy. some people might prefer to take medication at home rather than ＿＿＿＿＿＿＿＿＿.

Other treatment options in addition to therapy and medication: (paras. 18-21)

Several studies have shown that ＿＿＿＿＿＿ may be helpful in managing mild to severe depression. For patients with more severe depression, ＿＿＿＿＿＿＿＿＿ and ＿＿＿＿＿＿＿＿＿ can be lifesaving treatments. Researchers are developing techniques including ＿＿＿＿＿＿＿＿＿ and ＿＿＿＿＿＿＿＿＿ to help guide decision-making. These technologies have shown promise, but they remain far from standard clinical practice.

Words and Phrases

I. Translate the following medical terms into Chinese or English.

1. side effect ＿＿＿＿＿＿＿＿＿＿＿＿＿＿＿＿

2. randomized trial ＿＿＿＿＿＿＿＿＿＿＿＿＿＿＿

3. evidence-based therapy ＿＿＿＿＿＿＿＿＿＿＿

4. medical circle ＿＿＿＿＿＿＿＿＿＿＿＿＿＿＿＿

140

5. 医疗实践　　　　　＿＿＿＿＿＿＿＿＿＿＿＿＿＿＿＿＿＿＿＿＿＿＿

6. 选择性血清素再摄取抑制剂　＿＿＿＿＿＿＿＿＿＿＿＿＿＿＿＿＿＿＿＿＿

7. 经颅磁刺激技术　　　　＿＿＿＿＿＿＿＿＿＿＿＿＿＿＿＿＿＿＿＿＿＿＿

8. 电惊厥疗法　　　　　＿＿＿＿＿＿＿＿＿＿＿＿＿＿＿＿＿＿＿＿＿＿＿

✔ II. Fill in the blanks with the words or phrases given below. Change the form if necessary.

| conducive | prescribe | grapple | alleviate | accessibility |

1. The idea that clear waters and green mountains are as good as mountains of gold and silver is ＿＿＿＿＿＿＿＿ to the sustainable development of global and regional economies.

2. During these years of my college life, I learn to ＿＿＿＿＿＿＿＿ with many challenges with a positive attitude.

3. People are becoming aware of the toll their jobs take on them, and employers are exploring ways to ＿＿＿＿＿＿＿＿ the harmful effects of stress and overwork.

4. China will continue to share its experience with other countries and work for greater ＿＿＿＿＿＿＿＿ and affordability of COVID-19 vaccines in developing countries.

5. The doctor did a thorough examination and ＿＿＿＿＿＿＿＿ three months of physical therapy for my leg injury.

Sentence Translation

Translate the following sentences into Chinese or English.

1. The study found that both psychotherapies and antidepressants were more effective than a placebo in reducing depressive symptoms in blinded trials. However, there was no significant difference in effectiveness between these two treatments.

＿＿＿＿＿＿＿＿＿＿＿＿＿＿＿＿＿＿＿＿＿＿＿＿＿＿＿＿＿＿＿＿＿＿＿＿

＿＿＿＿＿＿＿＿＿＿＿＿＿＿＿＿＿＿＿＿＿＿＿＿＿＿＿＿＿＿＿＿＿＿＿＿

2. Psychotherapies, such as cognitive behavioral therapy (CBT) or psychodynamic therapy (a form of talk therapy that investigates the interplay between unconscious emotions and distressing symptoms), can span months and include several hour-long sessions, which is

too much for many individuals.

_____

_____

3. The crunched time and administrative demands of modern medical practice sometimes result in rushed patient appointments that are more conducive to efficiency and medication than to meaningful discussions.

_____

_____

4. 认知行为疗法（CBT）教患者如何改变可能加剧抑郁的消极思维、感觉和行为模式。

_____

_____

5. 在医生出诊时增加检查项目可能会忽略治疗抑郁症的根本问题：我们是否分配了足够的时间与病人进行有意义的对话，让他们了解自己可做出的选择？

_____

_____

Text B

Pre-reading Questions:

1. How do you cheer yourself up when you feel upset?

2. How can you play a valuable role in supporting someone who suffers from emotional problems?

Easy Ways to Enhance Your Emotional Well-being

Text B

1. If you were hoping for a year of relative peace after the tumult of 2020 and 2021, you may have been disappointed. Natural catastrophes, worrying shortages, a new virus, a war in Europe, and the pandemic all stoked anxiety. However, there was also a lot of new information and understanding in 2022.

2. We discovered fresh ways to deal with life's stresses and build our mental resilience. These are a few of our favorite stories about mental health from the year, complete with crucial advice to usher you into a new year.

To Avoid Burnout, Be Aware of Its Physical Manifestations

3. There are several indications that your body may be experiencing burnout, such as sleeplessness, exhaustion, headaches, stomachaches, and changes in appetite. Although "burnout" may not be officially recognized as a medical condition, it is important not to disregard its symptoms, as documented by Melinda Wenner Moyer. Experts suggest that addressing burnout may need more than just indulging in self-care activities like bubble baths and cups of tea. It is advisable to seek guidance from a health care practitioner or a mental health professional in order to identify and address the underlying cause of the problem.

Comprehend the Distinctions between Burnout and Depression

4. It might be difficult to differentiate between burnout and depressive symptoms. Either one might make it hard for you to concentrate or lead to irregular or excessive sleep patterns.

Dani Blum claimed that burnout cannot be a diagnosable medical condition, but depression can.

5. Burnout may result in a sense of being overwhelmed by unrelenting work demands, leading to emotions of cynicism, depletion, and hatred towards one's profession. This can then result in a lack of energy for personal activities. According to Jeanette M. Bennett, an associate professor at the University of North Carolina at Charlotte who specializes in studying the impact of stress on health, individuals experiencing depression may not get any pleasure from their usual activities. Alternatively, you may choose to seclude yourself or disregard your personal hygiene and physical well-being. Gaining comprehension of the distinction is the first stage in discovering alleviation.

Discover Pleasure in Your Workouts

6. Imagine a moment when you were completely carefree and elated. Have you ever been to a concert and been all bouncing around? Whose sports team were you rooting for? It turns out that our own bodily expressions of happiness might, in turn, help us feel happier. A health psychologist and Stanford University professor named Kelly McGonigal created this eight-and-a-half-minute Joy Workout. It consists of six motions that are meant to make you happy, regardless of your age or ability level. The size and speed of your movements are entirely up to you. Although the exercise is shown standing up, you are free to experiment with sitting down, working out with friends or family, in or out of the house, and to whatever kind of music you choose.

An End to "Task Paralysis" Is within Your Reach

7. When you're overwhelmed, it's normal to freeze up; after all, what with all the things on your to-do list at home and the ever-increasing amount of work at your desk, it's often hard to know where to begin. According to Dana G. Smith, this is known as task paralysis, and it happens when your brain perceives your to-do list as a danger. And perfectionists are especially susceptible. Do not allow yourself to keep avoiding or putting things off if you want to nip this kind of anxiety in the bud. You may get a head start on the upcoming duties by reminding yourself of their importance and by giving yourself little prizes when you do them. Separating large projects into tangible steps may also be helpful. It will not

seem so daunting when you have considered the real amount of effort and time needed to complete the tasks.

Seek Solace in Nature's Soothing Embrace

8. There is an increasing amount of research indicating that engaging in activities in wilderness and environment, sometimes known as "ecotherapy," has many positive effects on mental health. Alisha Haridasani Gupta observed that engaging in activities such as hiking, white-water rafting, strolling on a tree-lined boulevard, or keeping a plant at home may all contribute to positive mental health outcomes. However, for many individuals, actually going outdoors might be more challenging than just expressing the intention to do so. Individuals of Black, Hispanic, and Asian descent have a threefold higher likelihood of residing in places that lack access to natural environments compared to individuals of white ethnicity. "Ms. Haridasani Gupta reported that even though natural spaces in the United States, such as national parks, are awe-inspiring, they are also tarnished with racist pasts." Across the nation, groups and discussion boards have emerged to promote outdoor recreation as a means for people of color to overcome mental health issues.

Learn the Steps to take in the Event of a Panic Attack

9. For those who have never been through one, panic attacks may be a terrifying experience. Dani Blum gave us a rundown of what panic attacks are and how to recognize them, which might include symptoms like a racing heart, a tight chest, nausea, tingly limbs, and a sensation as if you can't breathe. Additionally, she went over several self-coaching techniques, such as calming yourself by telling yourself you are not in danger, breathing deeply from your diaphragm, and contacting a friend for support. You may also find success with distraction activities, such as identifying the colors in your environment or counting to ten. If you've never had a panic attack before but are suddenly feeling chest discomfort and difficulty breathing, it's important to visit an emergency department to establish that you are not encountering a cardiac problem.

Learn about a Nerve That Is Vital to Your Health

10. The vagus nerve, sometimes called an "information superhighway," impacts almost every

internal organ as it travels from the brain to the belly. Many people on social media tout it as a key to tamping down anxiety, and claim it may assist with nervous system regulation, and relaxation, according to Christina Caron's report. In order to control the vagus nerve, some specialists recommend doing simple activities like timing your breathing or practicing mindfulness. Submerging your face in ice water may help you relax, according to some reports. This is because it activates the "diving reflex," which causes your heart rate to decrease and your blood vessels to constrict. Nevertheless, wellness entrepreneurs have also capitalized on this trend by offering goods such as "vagus massage oil," vibrating wristbands, and pillow mists, which lack scientific support.

Brown Noise Can Help You Relax and Unwind

11. According to Dani Blum, the deep and soothing hum of brown noise, which is comparable to white noise but has a lower pitch, is becoming more popular on the internet, particularly among those with attention-deficit/hyperactivity disorder. According to some individuals, brown noise has the ability to induce feelings of calmness, improve concentration, and reduce tension. On the other hand, other people find that brown noise helps them fall asleep more easily. However, for some individuals, the continuous sound of brown noise may be bothersome or anxiety provoking. According to experts, listening to brown noise for long durations is unlikely to cause damage (unless it is played at harmful levels). However, there is little evidence to suggest any good effects of doing so. If the rumbly sound of brown noise provides you tranquility, feel free to listen as often as you like.

Make the Most of Your Anxiety

12. Christina Caron said that although anxiousness may be debilitating when it spirals out of control, it can be a strength when it's under control. A healthy dose of worry might make you more careful and conscientious about potential dangers in your actions. Anxiety may be a symptom that something is wrong with your life and that you need to make a change. You may overcome your worries and develop inner strength by accepting your anxiousness.

First Things First: Identify Your Health "Non-Negotiables"

13. Dani Blum observed that little routines such as having a daily pastry with coffee and the

newspaper, or having a 90-pound Bernedoodle sitting in your lap, are what help us stay motivated and continue with our everyday lives. In this article, we invited readers to tell us about the daily rituals that sustain and enrich their lives. Some could ring a bell, or they might motivate you to start doing something different.

New Words and Expressions

New Words and
Expressions

tumult /ˈtjuːmʌlt/ *n.* a confused situation in which there is usually a lot of noise and excitement, often involving large numbers of people 骚乱；骚动；混乱；喧哗

stoke /stəʊk/ *v.* to make people feel sth. more strongly 煽动；激起

resilience /rɪˈzɪliəns/ *n.* the ability of people or things to feel better quickly after sth. unpleasant, such as shock, injury, etc. 快速恢复的能力；适应力

usher /ˈʌʃə(r)/ *v.* to take or show sb. where they should go 把……引往；引导；引领

diagnosable /daɪəɡˈnəʊzəbl/ *adj.* possible to diagnose 可诊断的

unrelenting /ˌʌnrɪˈlentɪŋ/ *adj.* not stopping or becoming less severe 持续的；不缓和的；势头不减的

cynicism /ˈsɪnɪsɪzəm/ *n.* an inclination to believe that people are motivated purely by self-interest; skepticism 愤世嫉俗；怀疑

depletion /dɪˈpliːʃn/ *n.* to reduce sth. by a large amount so that there is not enough left 大量减少；耗尽；使枯竭

hygiene /ˈhaɪdʒiːn/ *n.* the practice of keeping yourself and your living and working areas clean in order to prevent illness and disease 卫生

workout /ˈwɜːkaʊt/ *n.* a period of physical exercise that you do to keep fit 锻炼

elated /iˈleɪtɪd/ *adj.* very happy and excited because of sth. good that has happened or will happen 兴高采烈的；欢欣鼓舞的；喜气洋洋的

paralysis /pəˈræləsɪs/ *n.* a total inability to move, act, function, etc. (活动、工作等)能力的完全丧失；瘫痪

freeze up to suddenly become unable to think clearly or act effectively, often due to fear, anxiety, or stress 僵住；陷入困境

susceptible /səˈseptəbl/ *adj.* very likely to be influenced, harmed or affected by sb./sth. 易受影响(或伤害等)

nip sth. in the bud to stop a problem or issue before it becomes worse or more difficult to deal with 将……扼杀在萌芽状态；防患于未然

tangible /ˈtændʒəbl/ *adj.* that can be clearly seen to exist 有形的；实际的；真实的

daunting /ˈdɔːntɪŋ/ *adj.* discouraging through fear 令人畏惧的；使人气馁的；令人却步的

ecotherapy /ˌiːkəʊˈθerəpi/ *n.* therapy that covers a host of natural treatments 生态疗法

white-water rafting the activity of riding on a raft over rough, dangerous parts of a fast-flowing river 乘竹筏漂流

awe-inspiring /ˈɔːɪnˈspaɪərɪŋ/ *adj.* impressive; making you feel respect and admiration 令人惊叹的；使人敬佩的；令人敬慕的

tarnish /ˈtɑːnɪʃ/ *v.* to spoil the good opinion people have of sb./sth. 玷污；败坏；损坏(名声等)

tingly /ˈtɪŋɡli/ *adj.* causing or experiencing a slight feeling of tingling 引起(或感到)轻微刺痛的

limb /lɪm/ *n.* an arm or a leg; a similar part of an animal, such as a wing 肢；臂；腿；翼；翅膀

diaphragm /ˈdaɪəfræm/ *n.* the layer of muscle between the lungs and the stomach, used especially to control breathing 膈；膈膜；横膈膜

cardiac /ˈkɑːdiæk/ *adj.* connected with the heart or heart disease 心脏的；心脏病的

nerve /nɜːv/ *n.* any of the long threads that carry messages between the brain and parts of the body, enabling you to move, feel pain, etc. 神经

vagus /ˈveɪɡəs/ *n.* a mixed nerve that supplies the pharynx and larynx and lungs and heart and esophagus and stomach and most of the abdominal viscera 迷走神经

tout /taʊt/ *v.* to try to persuade people that sb./sth. is important or valuable by praising them/it 标榜；吹捧；吹嘘

tamp /tæmp/ *v.* press down tightly 压低

submerge /səbˈmɜːdʒ/ v. to go under the surface of water or liquid; to put sth. or make sth. go under the surface of water or liquid (使)潜入水中；没入水中；浸没；淹没

reflex /ˈriːfleks/ n. an action or a movement of your body that happens naturally in response to sth. and that you cannot control; sth. that you do without thinking 反射动作；本能反应；反射作用

blood vessel any of the tubes through which blood flows through the body 血管

constrict /kənˈstrɪkt/ v. to become tighter or narrower; to make sth. tighter or narrower (使)紧缩；缩窄

capitalize /ˈkæpɪtəlaɪz/ v. to sell possessions in order to change them into money 变现

soothing /suːðɪŋ/ adj. freeing from fear and anxiety 慰藉的；使人宽心的；镇静的

hum /hʌm/ n. a low continuous sound 嗡嗡声；嘈杂声

hyperactivity /ˌhaɪpərækˈtɪvətɪ/ n. a condition characterized by excessive restlessness and movement 活动过度；极度活跃

provoking /prəˈvəʊkɪŋ/ adj. causing or tending to cause 刺激的

rumbly /ˈrʌmblɪ/ adj. tending to rumble or rattle 发隆隆声的

debilitating /dɪˈbɪlɪteɪtɪŋ/ adj. impairing the strength and vitality 使(人或人的身体)非常虚弱的

spiral /ˈspaɪrəl/ v. to increase rapidly 急剧增长

conscientious /ˌkɒnʃiˈenʃəs/ adj. taking care to do things carefully and correctly 勤勉认真的；一丝不苟的

pastry /ˈpeɪstri/ n. any of various baked foods made of dough or batter 糕点

🔲 Notes

1. vagus nerve: A mixed nerve that supplies the pharynx and larynx and lungs and heart and esophagus and stomach and most of the abdominal viscera.

迷走神经是供应咽、喉、肺、心脏、食管、胃和大部分腹部内脏的混合神经。

2. brown noise: Brown noise is a type of low-frequency sound produced by the same

process that causes Brownian motion. It has nothing to do with color; instead, brown noise gets its name from the 19th-century Scottish botanist Robert Brown, who discovered a certain kind of random microscopic motion that is now referred to as Brownian motion.

布朗噪声是由引起布朗运动的相同过程产生的一种低频声音。它与颜色无关；相反，布朗噪声的名字来源于 19 世纪的苏格兰植物学家罗伯特·布朗，他发现了一种随机的微观运动，现在被称为"布朗运动"。

3. attention-deficit/hyperactivity disorder：Attention-deficit/hyperactivity disorder（ADHD）is a behavioral disorder that typically begins in childhood and is characterized by a short attention span, an inability to be calm and stay still, and poor impulse control.

注意缺陷多动障碍（ADHD）是一种行为障碍，通常始于儿童时期，其特征是注意力持续时间短、无法平静和静止以及冲动控制能力差。

4. Bernedoodle：The Bernedoodle is a cross between a Bernese Mountain Dog and a Poodle.

伯尔尼多德尔是伯恩山犬和贵宾犬的混血品种。

▤ After Reading Activities

Reading Comprehension

Decide whether the following statements are true (T) or false (F) according to the text.

_____ 1. With burnout, you might not find your hobbies enjoyable at all.

_____ 2. It is true that the actions we take in response to happiness can also trigger feelings of happiness.

_____ 3. Perfectionists are particularly prone to experiencing anxiety for having too many tasks.

_____ 4. If you are experiencing chest pain and shortness of breath, you have a panic attack.

_____ 5. Vibrating bracelets and pillow mists are effective products for helping people calm down.

Words and Phrases

Match each English phrase in Column A with its Chinese version in Column B.

Column A	Column B
1. associate professor	A. 心理韧性
2. vagus nerve	B. 布朗噪声
3. blood vessel	C. 迷走神经
4. brown noise	D. 医护人员
5. panic attack	E. 身体状况
6. medical condition	F. 惊恐发作
7. health care practitioner	G. 副教授
8. mental resilience	H. 血管

Translation

开始接受高等教育是年轻人人生的一个关键转折点。这是一个经常伴随着重大变化的阶段，夹杂着学生对大学生活的高期望，以及他们自己和他人对学习成绩的高期望。相关因素包括离开家庭、学会独立生活、发展新的社交网络、适应新的学习方式，以及还要应对额外的更大的经济负担。高等教育机构有一个独特的机会来识别、预防和治疗学生的心理健康问题，因为它们在学生生活的多个方面提供支持，包括学术学习、娱乐活动、咨询服务和住宿。

_____

_____

_____

_____

Critical Thinking

If one of your friends experiences severe anxiety due to the immense pressure at college, how will you communicate with him or her? Please work in groups to have a discussion focusing on suggestions for dealing with the anxiety and seeking appropriate help.

Part III　Apply Medical English

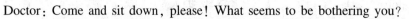

Dialogue

A. Situational Dialogues in Different Clinical Departments

Ophthalmology(眼科)

Conjunctivitis(结膜炎)

Doctor：Come and sit down, please! What seems to be bothering you?

Patient：I think there's something wrong with my eyes. I found that my eyes were red a week ago. And now they are getting worse.

Doctor：Do you have any other symptoms? Did you feel itches in your eyes?

Patient：Sometimes. And I have a foreign body sensation in my eyes every now and then, so I can't help rubbing my eyes.

Doctor：Do you see objects dimly?

Patient：No. It seems my sight is not affected.

Doctor：Do you live with others? Has anyone else in the house had a similar problem?

Patient：Yes, I live with my parents. My mother seems to have similar but milder symptoms.

Doctor：OK. Try not to blink. I'll give you an examination.

Patient：Sure. What am I suffering from? Is it serious?

Doctor：Don't worry. It is conjunctivitis. It can be cured by some simple therapies.

Patient：It's nice to hear that! What should I do?

Doctor：I will give you a prescription. Use the eye drops four times a day. And come back here for a check in two weeks. There's one more important thing. Because conjunctivitis is highly contagious, you cannot share handkerchiefs, tissues, towels, cosmetics, or bedsheets with uninfected family or friends. Also, hand washing is an essential and highly effective way to prevent the spread of infection.

Patient：OK. Thank you, doctor!

📋 Words and Phrases

itch /ɪtʃ/ *n.* 痒

foreign body sensation /ˈfɒrən ˈbɒdi senˈseɪʃn/ *n.* 异物感

dimly /ˈdɪmli/ *adv.* 模糊地

milder /ˈmaɪldə/ *adj.* 更轻微的

conjunctivitis /kənˌdʒʌŋktɪˈvaɪtɪs/ *n.* 结膜炎

eye drop /aɪ drɒp/ *n.* 滴眼剂

📋 Notes

Eye diseases

Eye diseases are conditions that affect any part of your eyes, and include conditions that affect the structures immediately around your eyes. These conditions can be acute (meaning they develop quickly) or chronic (meaning they develop more slowly and last a long time). Your eyeball itself is where most eye diseases happen, but it isn't the only place. Eye diseases also include conditions that can affect your eye muscles, eye socket, eyelids, or the skin and muscles immediately around your eyes.

Here are some most common eye diseases worldwide.

Refractive errors

Refractive errors are the most frequent eye problems in the world. They include: myopia (nearsightedness), hyperopia (farsightedness), astigmatism (distorted vision at all distances), presbyopia that occurs between age 40-50 years (loss of the ability to focus up close, inability to read words in a book, need to hold newspaper farther away to see clearly). Refractive errors can be corrected by eyeglasses, contact lenses, or in some cases surgery.

Age-related macular degeneration

Age-related macular degeneration (AMD) results in damaged sharp and central vision. Central vision is needed for seeing objects clearly and for reading and driving. AMD affects the macula, the central part of the retina that allows the eye to see fine details.

Cataract

Cataract is a clouding of the eye's lens. It's the leading cause of blindness worldwide. It can occur at any age and can be present at birth. Removing cataracts is a widely available treatment.

Glaucoma

Glaucoma is a group of diseases that can damage the eye's optic nerve and result in vision loss and blindness. Glaucoma occurs when the normal fluid pressure inside the eyes slowly rises. However, recent findings show that glaucoma can occur with normal eye pressure. With early treatment, you can often protect your eyes against serious vision loss.

Amblyopia

Amblyopia is the most common cause of vision impairment in children. With amblyopia, the vision in one eye is reduced because the eye and the brain are not working together properly. The eye itself looks normal, but it is not being used normally because the brain is favoring the other eye.

眼病是指影响眼睛任何部位的疾病，包括影响眼睛周围结构的疾病。这些情况可以是急性的（意味着它们发展得很快），也可以是慢性的（意味着它们发展得更慢，持续时间更长）。眼球本身是大多数眼病发生的地方，但它并不是唯一的地方。眼部疾病还包括可能影响眼睛肌肉、眼窝、眼睑或眼睛周围皮肤和肌肉的疾病。

以下是一些最常见的眼病。

屈光不正

屈光不正是世界上最常见的眼部问题。它们包括：近视、远视、散光（所有距离的视力扭曲）、年龄在 40~50 岁之间的患者所得的老花眼（失去近距离聚焦的能力，无法阅读书中的词，需要把报纸拿得更远才能看清楚）。屈光不正可以通过眼镜、隐形眼镜或在某些情况下进行手术来矫正。

老年性黄斑变性

老年性黄斑变性（AMD）会导致视物变形和中心视力受损。中心视力是清晰观察物体、阅读和驾驶所必需的。老年性黄斑变性会影响在视网膜中央部分的能让眼睛看到细节的黄斑。

白内障

白内障是指眼睛晶状体变混浊。它是全世界范围内失明的主要原因。白内障可发生在任何年龄，也可能在出生时就存在。摘除白内障是一种广泛使用的治疗方法。

青光眼

青光眼是一种可损害眼睛视神经并导致视力下降和失明的疾病。当眼球内的正常液体压力缓慢升高时，就会发生青光眼。然而，最近的研究结果表明，正常眼压也会导致青光眼。如果及早治疗，眼睛通常可以得到保护，避免视力严重下降。

弱视

弱视是儿童视力障碍的最常见原因。弱视是指一只眼睛与大脑的协调不正常而导致视力降低。这只眼睛本身看起来正常，但由于大脑偏爱另一只眼睛，因而未被正常使用。

▤ Practical Activity

Work with your partner to create and perform a doctor-patient dialogue related to eye diseases.

✅ B. Practical Unit Project

Please work in pairs to create and role-play a conversation between a doctor in psychiatry and a college student who has psychological problems.

Guidance for Production

Tips for making a conversation：

Step 1：Brainstorm your ideas and write them down.

- Why does the student feel depressed?
- How does the doctor check him/her?
- What suggestions does the doctor make?
- Does the doctor prescribe any medication?
- How can the student get the medication?

Step 2：Write an outline.

The outline will help make your ideas clearer and to the point.

Step 3：Create and revise your conversation.

When you begin to create your conversation, try to use words, phrases and sentence patterns you have learned from this unit.

Step 4：Rehearse in pairs.

Try to be as natural and fluent as you can.

Part IV Self-Assessment

Use the following self-assessment checklist to check what you have learned in this unit.

I understand the basic concept of psychological treatment.	☐
I can identify and use the words, phrases and sentence patterns related to the topic.	☐
I can make a conversation by using the terminologies and medical information in this unit with my partner.	☐
I can embrace future life with a positive attitude.	☐

Unit 6
Doctor-Patient Communication

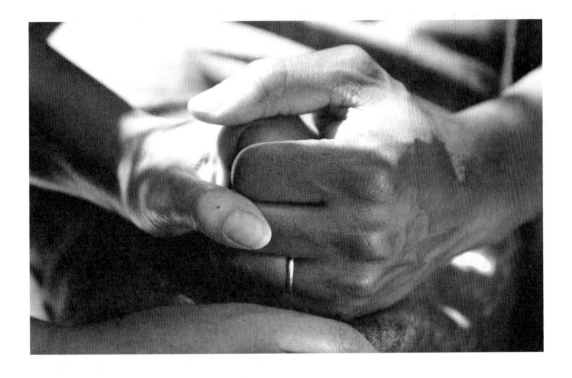

Doctor-patient communication is a complex topic between a doctor and a patient in the process of health care. It is conducted but not confined to when a doctor attends to a patient's medical needs. In a good doctor-patient communication, the doctor trusts the patient to reveal any information that may be relevant to the case and in turn, the patient trusts the doctor to respect their privacy and not disclose this information to outside parties. In more recent times, health care has become more patient-centered and this has brought a new dynamic to this ancient topic. The quality of the doctor-patient

Lead in

157

communication is important to both parties. An effective and efficient communication between the doctor and patient will lead to frequent, quality information about the patient's disease and better health care for the patient and their family.

This unit is mainly to achieve the following objectives:

1) Understand the impact of doctor-patient communication in health care;

2) Identify words, phrases and sentence patterns related to the topic;

3) Write an essay by using the terminologies and medical information in this unit;

4) Learn the importance and skills of maintaining a good doctor-patient communication.

Part I   View the Medical World

Watch a video about doctor-patient communication and choose the right answer.①

1. What is the video's intended purpose?

    A. To show us ways to deal with angry and upset patients.

    B. To teach us to show sympathy to angry and upset doctors.

    C. To show us a way to pay our respect to doctors.

    D. To show us the importance of talking effectively and efficiently.

2. According to Dr. Drummond, there are _____ steps of in the Universal Upset Person Protocol.

    A. 6   B. 5   C. 4   D. 3

3. _____ is the first thing to do when dealing with an upset person.

    A. Talking about what brought them in

    B. Talking about the weather

    C. Helping them understand what they're really feeling

    D. Sharing their love stories and family life

4. _____ does not belong to the Universal Upset Person Protocol.

    A. Telling the patients that they look really upset

    B. Telling the patients to share their stories

    C. Telling the patients to yell out loud their pains

    D. Telling the patients you feel sorry for their sufferings

5. For a doctor, _____ is critically important to maintaining bond with this patient.

    A. being polite

    B. loving their stories

    C. knowing the importance of good health

    D. showing that you have sympathy for their situation

---

① 视频详见网站:https://pan-yz. cldisk. com/external/m/file/1055138621237186560。

📑 Words and Phrases

ambushed /ˈæmbʊʃt/ *adj.* 中埋伏的

protocol /ˈprəʊtəkɒl/ *n.* 协议；议定书

throw gas on a fire /θrəʊ gæs ɒn ə ˈfaɪə(r) / 火上浇油

vent /vent/ *v.* 表达；发泄(感情，尤指愤怒)

get clear on /get klɪə(r) ɒn / 弄清楚

breeze through /briːz θruː/ 轻松地做某事

Part II　Read to Explore Medical Knowledge

Text A

Pre-reading Questions:

1. To what extent does the pandemic change the doctor-patient relationship?

2. Why is communication between physician and patients often disrupted or completely cut?

Effective Doctor-Patient Communication: The Foundation of Quality Health Care

Text A

1. It is expected that the doctor and patient would communicate with each other. It is essential for diagnosis, treatment, and, likely, recovery. In light of the fact that the digital revolution is radically altering the relationship between patients and health care providers, what should the nature of communication be in order to establish a reliable therapeutic doctor-patient relationship?

2. The subject has been covered extensively in both scholarly and popular publications. Just ask Dr. Google, and he'll pull up a plethora of papers titled "The Importance of Doctor-Patient Communication," "How Can Doctors Improve Their Communication Skills in Health Care?" and numerous more.

3. Nevertheless, it has come to my attention from my interactions with health care professionals (HCPs) over the years that it is doubtful these papers are truly read. I've encountered physicians who rarely look into the patient's eyes, who cut you off in the middle of your speech, who prescribe prescriptions without properly diagnosing the condition or asking about potential side effects, who never follow up with test results, and so on.

4. I was able to navigate the health care provider's mumblings, the infamous Dr. Google, and the pharmacist's instructions, so it didn't really annoy me.

5. The significance of clear, concise, and empathetic communication between patients and their health care providers was brought to my attention when I received an unexpected breast cancer diagnosis. Imagine if it could mitigate the perception of a potentially fatal diagnosis into an unexpectedly beneficial educational opportunity, thereby easing the burden brought by the diagnosis and the adverse effects of the treatment, and making the patient's adherence to therapy easier. It was not only the in-person interactions I had with doctors and nurses that made getting a diagnosis, undergoing surgery, and recovering from treatment much easier; what transpired in the meantime also played a role in maintaining my unfaltering conviction that "we" could triumph over this challenge.

6. These features encompass a wealth of information, including extensive reading materials sent to my inbox to supplement and broaden the knowledge I gained during in-person consultations, an accessible email channel and brief messaging system where members of the treatment team responded quickly to my questions, timely appointment reminders, alerts when appointments were running late, and even a virtual meeting with my oncologist after hours when an appointment had to be canceled due to an emergency on her end.

Results of Ineffective Communication

7. It might be challenging for patients to establish a trustworthy and meaningful relationship with their treatment team as I did. Many factors contribute to the breakdown of physician-patient communication. These include an overwhelming amount of administrative work, concerns about litigation, patients' unrealistic expectations, and a lack of emphasis on communication skills during medical school. As a result, patients are dissatisfied and may lack compliance with treatment, which in turn can lead to poor clinical outcomes and, in the worst-case scenario, malpractice lawsuits.

8. More than half of medication errors, which frequently result in negative outcomes or even death, were caused by a lack of communication between patients and their doctors or between prescribing doctors and other members of the health care team, according to statistics cited during a recent webinar on the topic. One of the most common reasons individuals choose to sue for medical malpractice is because of misunderstanding on the part

of physicians and other medical staff.

9. What's more, when people believe their doctor isn't communicating well with them, it may have devastating effects on the doctor's practice and reputation. This includes unhappy patients who won't come back and bad reviews that can make it hard for the doctor to get new patients.

10. The literature on effective or ineffective patient-physician contact emphasizes that the key elements are patients' perceptions of the encounter, the degree of doctors' empathy, and the doctors' communication style, tone of voice, and non-verbal cues.

The Influence of Technology

11. Gone are the days when people would just accept their diagnosis and treatment plan. Patients now have the authority and basic knowledge to demand answers from Dr. Google, despite the fact that he frequently makes mistakes or is misinterpreted.

12. Furthermore, the COVID-19 pandemic has brought about a shift in the conventional face-to-face patient-physician contact to virtual communication. Since patients and physicians are physically separated, telemedicine technology needs to advance quickly to provide consultations. This raises a number of ethical concerns but also presents a myriad of potential to enhance and broaden communication channels.

13. Pallavi Bradshaw of the MPS wonders aloud in an editorial piece published in the *BMJ* whether the pandemic has irrevocably altered the doctor-patient relationship. Bradshaw writes that the answer is "yes", but that there is a heightened chance of misunderstandings and incorrect diagnoses when medical examinations are restricted.

14. Nevertheless, she clarifies that these dangers can be "at least partially reduced" by changing the way we engage with clients, which includes listening more attentively, reviewing previous material, and using a pleasant tone. Telemedicine will continue to play an important role due to its low cost, high convenience, and low risk; however, it may potentially be detrimental to our relationship with patients.

15. Preliminary research has shown that particularly younger patients prefer technologically savvy health care providers who can communicate with them through the communication channels they are using in their daily life such as texting, video and voice calls. Automated text messages such as reminders of appointments and preventative and pre-appointment

requirements such as fasting have been proven to be highly effective, while apps that allow patients to view their medical history empower them to become active participants in their care.

16. New patient relationship management (PRM) systems provide innovative ways to maintain open communication channels between patients and health care providers. These systems optimize and support patients throughout their care journey, facilitate information flow within health care systems, and make it easier to start, track, and record conversations.

Revisiting Communication Proficiency

17. To deal with potential miscommunication problems, there needs to be a renewed focus on the fundamentals of good doctor-patient communication, whether it happens in person or online.

18. A lack of insight due to inadequate knowledge and training in communication, doctors often not understanding the importance of keeping patients adequately informed, and failure to pay attention to non-verbal components of the communication are some of the main barriers to good health care communication, according to an article published in the *Journal of Clinical and Diagnostic Research*. Furthermore, communication breakdowns may be caused by stress, exhaustion, and a lack of time, especially in a health care facility that is already overcrowded.

19. Advice on good communication in health care by the authors includes:

- Exhibit patience and attentiveness towards both the spoken and unspoken aspects of the patient's communication. It is important for doctors to watch their own body language, gestures, eye contact, and vocal intonation as well as those of their patients. Although studies have demonstrated that nonverbal communication does affect patient satisfaction, it is generally regarded as less significant.

- Show interest in talking to patients through mannerisms, body language, and active involvement, such as leaning towards them.

- Listen carefully and be sure not to interrupt when the patient is telling something.

- Always offer helpful information when necessary and quickly respond to the patient's reaction. Articles, brochures, and FAQs should be provided in case serious and chronic diseases are diagnosed.

- Discuss the disease's nature, course, prognosis, treatment options, and the need for investigations.

- Discuss the necessity and feasibility of expensive investigations and drugs and their effect on main course and outcome of disease.

- Get the patient involved in the decision-making. The treatment plan must conform to the patient's cognition.

- Put extra effort into encouraging patients' adherence to lifestyle changes.

- Use simple language instead of medical jargon.

Conclusion

20. The rapid digital transformation in health care has stimulated huge debates on the possible risks and ethical concerns, but there is no turning back. Health care professionals must adjust and acquire the skills to minimize the potential hazards of digital communication with their patients. They should adhere to the conventional principles of empathy, truthfulness, and respect in order to gather accurate information, facilitate precise diagnosis and treatment, and ultimately provide high-quality care and positive outcomes.

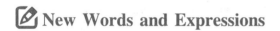 **New Words and Expressions**

New Words and
Expressions

therapeutic /ˌθerəˈpjuːtɪk/ *adj.* designed to help treat an illness 治疗的；医疗的

navigate /ˈnævɪgeɪt/ *v.* to find the right way to deal with a difficult or complicated situation 找到正确方法(对付困难复杂的情况)

mumbling /ˈmʌmblɪŋ/ *n.* speech or words that are spoken in a quiet voice in a way that is not clear 喃喃自语；嘟哝

infamous /ˈɪnfəməs/ *adj.* well known for being bad or evil 臭名远扬的；声名狼藉的

pharmacist /ˈfɑːməsɪst/ *n.* a person whose job is to prepare medicines and sell or give them to the public in a shop/store or in a hospital 药剂师

empathetic /ˌempəˈθetɪk/ *adj.* involving, characterized by, or based on empathy 移情的；有同感的；能产生共鸣的

mitigate /ˈmɪtɪgeɪt/ *v.* to make sth. less harmful, serious, etc. 减轻；缓和

perception /pəˈsepʃn/ *n.* the ability to understand the true nature of sth. 洞察力；悟性

adherence /ədˈhɪərəns/ *n.* the fact of behaving according to a particular rule, etc., or of following a particular set of beliefs, or a fixed way of doing sth. 坚持；遵守；遵循

unfaltering /ˌʌnˈfɔːltərɪŋ/ *adj.* marked by firm determination or resolution 坚决的

consultation /ˌkɒnslˈteɪʃn/ *n.* a meeting with an expert, especially a doctor, to get advice or treatment（向专家请教的）咨询会；（尤指）就诊

oncologist /ɒŋˈkɒlədʒist/ *n.* a specialist in oncology 肿瘤专家

administrative /ədˈmɪnɪstrətɪv/ *adj.* connected with organizing the work of a business or an institution 管理的；行政的

litigation /ˌlɪtɪˈgeɪʃn/ *n.* the process of making or defending a claim in court 诉讼；打官司

compliance /kəmˈplaɪəns/ *n.* the practice of obeying rules or requests made by people in authority 服从；顺从；遵从

scenario /səˈnɑːriəʊ/ *n.* a description of how things might happen in the future 方案；预测

malpractice /ˌmælˈpræktɪs/ *v.* careless, wrong or illegal behavior while in a professional job 玩忽职守

prescribing doctor a health care professional who is authorized to write prescriptions for medications and other treatments 开处方的医生

webinar /ˈwebɪnɑː(r)/ *n.* a seminar that is conducted over the internet 在线研讨会

empathy /ˈempəθi/ *n.* the ability to understand another person's feelings, experience, etc. 同感；共鸣；同情

telemedicine /telɪˈmedɪsən/ *n.* medical care provided remotely to a patient in a separate location using two-way voice and visual communication（as by computer or cell phone）远程医疗

myriad /ˈmɪriəd/ *n.* an extremely large number of sth. 无数；大量

heighten /ˈhaɪtn/ *v.* if a feeling or an effect heightens, or sth. heightens it, it becomes stronger or increases（使）加强；提高；增加

detrimental /ˌdetrɪˈmentl/ *adj.* harmful 有害的；不利的

preliminary /prɪˈlɪmɪnəri/ *adj.* happening before a more important action or event 预备性的；初步的；开始的

savvy /ˈsævi/ *adj.* practical knowledge or understanding of sth. 有见识的

fasting /ˈfɑːstɪŋ/ *n.* a period during which you do not eat food, especially for religious or health reasons 禁食期；斋戒期

optimize /ˈɒptɪmaɪz/ *v.* to make sth. as good as it can be; to use sth. in the best possible way 使最优化；充分利用

revisit /ˌriːˈvɪzɪt/ *v.* to return to an idea or a subject and discuss it again 重提；再次讨论

mannerism /ˈmænərɪzəm/ *n.* a particular habit or way of speaking or behaving that sb. has but is not aware of 习性；言谈举止

brochure /ˈbrəʊʃə(r)/ *n.* a small magazine or book containing pictures and information about sth. or advertising sth. 资料(或广告)手册

prognosis /prɒɡˈnəʊsɪs/ *n.* an opinion, based on medical experience, of the likely development of a disease or an illness(对病情的)预断；预后

feasibility /ˌfiːzəˈbɪlɪti/ *n.* the quality of being doable 可能性；可行性

conform /kənˈfɔːm/ *v.* to behave and think in the same way as most other people in a group or society 顺从；顺应(大多数人或社会)；随潮流

jargon /ˈdʒɑːɡən/ *n.* words or expressions that are used by a particular profession or group of people, and are difficult for others to understand 行话；行业术语

🗒 Notes

1. Dr. Google: It is a humorous of way of saying the website Google, a search engine where people can type words in order to find information about sb. or sth.

这是一种幽默的说法，谷歌是一个搜索引擎，人们可以在这里输入单词来查找有关某人或某事的信息。

2. *BMJ*: The *British Medical Journal* is a leading medical journal that publishes original research, news, education, and opinion on various topics in health care.

《英国医学杂志》是一份领先的医学杂志，该杂志发表关于医疗保健各个主题的原创研究、新闻、教育文章和观点。

3. MPS: Abbreviation of Member of the Pharmaceutical Society. Parliament of

Pharmaceutical Society is a British group that determines the professional qualifications and enforces discipline for pharmacists.

　　MPS 是药剂师协会会员的缩写。药剂师协会是英国负责确定药剂师的专业资格并执行规章制度的协会。

📄 After Reading Activities

Reading Comprehension

✅ I. Answer the following questions.

1. What forced the author into realizing the importance of good doctor-patient communication?

2. How can effective communication help the doctors and patients?

3. What kind of damage can poor communication between doctors and patients lead to?

4. List some good communication skills mentioned in the passage.

5. How does communication between doctors and patients change before and after the COVID-19 pandemic?

✅ II. Work in groups to complete the following chart according to the structure of the text.

Concerns over doctor-patient relationship：(paras. 1-2)

　　Doctor-patient relationship has long been a popular topic. _____ about the topic are abundant.

My experience of encountering with health care professionals (paras. 3-6)

1. Interactions with health care professionals were brought to my attention _____ _____. (paras. 3-4)

2. An unexpected breast cancer diagnosis forced me into realizing _____ between health care professionals and the patient. (paras. 5-6)

My thoughts about doctor-patient communication during the process of treating breast cancer (paras. 7-19)

1. Results of ineffective communication (paras. 7-10)

　　Establishing _____ with health care professionals is by no means easy.

Consequences brought by poor communication are detrimental.

2. The influence of technology (paras. 11-16)

Many factors such as the help of Mr. Google, _____ etc. contribute to change our way of doctor-patient communication from face to face consultation to _____

_____.

3. Revisiting communication proficiency (paras. 17-19)

Suggestions to improve the effectiveness of doctor-patient communication are provided.

Conclusion: (para. 20)

Despite the great digital transformation, health care professionals should still adhere to _____ of empathy, truthfulness, and respect in order to provide high-quality care.

Words and Phrases

✅ I. Translate the following medical terms into Chinese or English.

1. effective communication between the doctor and patient   _____

2. establish a trustworthy and meaningful relationship   _____

3. poor clinical outcomes   _____

4. patients' unrealistic expectations   _____

5. 拓展沟通渠道   _____

6. 医护人员的喃喃自语   _____

7. 诊断及治疗方案   _____

8. 检查的可行性   _____

✅ II. Fill in the blanks with the words or phrases given below. Change the form if necessary.

mitigate	perception	unfaltering	empathy	consultation

1. He is interested in how our _____ of death affect the way we live.

2. Exercise to some degree could _____ the psychological stress reactions.

3. Given the remarkable contributions by our ancestors, I strongly believe that modern Chinese scientists can also make outstanding achievements through _____ patience and

persistent devotion.

4. The nurse's _____ manner made the anxious patient feel heard and understood, creating a comforting environment during the consultation.

5. A personal diet plan is devised after a _____ with a nutritionist.

Sentence Translation

Translate the following sentences into Chinese or English.

1. These systems optimize and support patients throughout their care journey, facilitate information flow within health care systems, and make it easier to start, track, and record conversations.

_____

_____

2. Since patients and physicians are physically separated, telemedicine technology needed to advance quickly to provide consultations. This raised a number of ethical concerns but also presented a myriad of potential to enhance and broaden communication channels.

_____

_____

3. Although studies have demonstrated that nonverbal communication does affect patient satisfaction, it is generally regarded as less significant than verbal communication.

_____

_____

4. 讨论昂贵的检查和药物的必要性和可行性及它们对主要病程和疾病结果的影响。

_____

_____

5. 医护人员必须调整和掌握沟通技巧，从而尽量减少与患者进行数字网络沟通的潜在风险。

_____

_____

Text B

Pre-reading Questions:

1. How do you think a person would react to their cancer diagnosis? To what extent would they agree to the doctor's treatment proposal?

2. Is it important for doctors to show empathy in patient care? Why?

Text B

Are You Listening?

Bond between Doctors and Patients is Challenged by Modern Medicine.

1. Kimberly Allison was able to accept her treatment plan following a sad diagnosis after talking to her oncology team.

2. The diagnosis was delivered to Kimberly Allison, M.D., at the age of 33. After a few weeks on the job, she was already settling into her new routine with her husband, preschool-aged daughter, and infant son at the University of Washington Medical Center's breast cancer pathology lab.

3. "Like Alice in Wonderland, falling down the rabbit hole" was the description of her reaction to learning that she had the illness she had spent her life researching.

4. The scientist couldn't help but notice that young women are more likely to have cancer, and that this type of cancer is often more lethal. Unconsciously, the cancer had become undetected and massive throughout her pregnancy and nursing.

5. Now as a professor of pathology at Stanford's School of Medicine, Allison remembers the "darkest places" she scoured for solutions during her severe depression following the diagnosis a decade ago.

6. "The results of every study I found were disastrous. It seemed like a death sentence to me," she adds. Now imagine you're down to your last two years. Go there immediately. How would you suggest she use that time? She felt an overwhelming sense of sadness for her children. Is it better if she takes time off to be with her spouse and children rather than

work? Is it more rewarding for her to write or paint? Alternatively, she might continue pursuing her passion for her job.

7. Until she met with her oncology team, she would not be able to put those worries to rest.

8. During her initial consultation with her surgeon and two oncologists, Allison willed emotion away. With the doctors congregating around the conference table beside her husband, she was afraid she would "be a total mess" if she did. The last thing she wanted was for her coworkers to doubt her competence or professionalism.

9. They discussed the cancer's symptoms and treatment options in a matter-of-fact way, and they came up with a plan: radiation first, then surgery, and finally six months of chemotherapy. The team could get to work immediately.

10. Allison, however, felt uneasy. "Alright, but I've seen the pathology," she informed the group. "I think this is terrible." At that moment, Kristine Calhoun, M.D., Allison's surgeon, recognized the terror hiding beneath Allison's tough facade. "I know you've looked up your prognosis," Calhoun told her. "However, this result is being altered with the advent of novel targeted medicines. The data is so new that it hasn't been included in the previous articles concerning malignancies connected with pregnancy."

11. "This is a whole new ballgame," remarked Calhoun. "Visiting the grandkids is what we're discussing."

12. Allison described her newfound hope as a "reset" that made her realize, "OK, I'm not dying."

13. Calhoun, who is currently a medical student at the University of Washington, emphasizes the importance of helping Allison see a positive future while stating that there is a fine line between offering patients hope and giving them false hope.

14. She claims that people who lose hope kind of will themselves into a certain pathway. The way Allison handled the situation taught Calhoun a lot, even if it was not always easy to treat a friend.

15. It made her more empathic, and she adds. "It taught me to see patients as more than just a diagnosis."

16. According to Stanford physician and author Abraham Verghese, M.D., the bond between Allison and Calhoun, which deepened throughout Allison's treatment, exemplifies the

"most poignant of human experiences"—the compassion for those who are suffering and the pain itself.

17. "The relationship between a care provider and a patient is vitally important in determining the health and well-being of the patient and the outcome of treatments," affirms Lloyd Minor, M.D., dean of the School of Medicine.

18. He points out that in the past, doctors could only provide solace to their sick patients by listening with compassion and understanding. Everything changed, and patient care improved significantly with the recent advancement of biological knowledge and treatment alternatives. However, he insists that in order to enhance doctors' ability to understand and care for their patients, it is necessary to address the "separation between the science of medicine and the humanism and compassion of medicine" that this purportedly caused.

19. According to Minor, "Every patient comes with a different history, with a different social, cultural and behavioral background. The efficacy of any treatments you hope to provide based on scientific evidence will depend significantly on those factors."

20. Minor, who instructed an undergraduate course on empathy, medicine, and literature last winter, believes that caregivers' well-being and a patient's motivation to recover are greatly improved when they perceive the support of the entire team. One of the many reasons being a doctor is a calling, in his words, is "interacting with people in a way that establishes deep personal relationships that are unique to health care".

21. New care models based on that type of trust are being developed by Alan Glaseroff, M.D., adjunct professor of medicine, and Arnold Milstein, M.D., professor of medicine and director of Stanford's Clinical Excellence Research Center.

22. The Stanford Coordinated Care program was founded in 2011 by Glaseroff and his wife, Ann Lindsay, M.D. They left Humboldt County to do this, drawing on their extensive experience in family practice in Arcata, California, and gleaned from their fifteen years of collaboration with the Institute of Health Care Improvement and other trailblazers in the national effort to reimagine primary care.

23. By focusing on the 5% of employees and their families whose care accounts for 50% of the plan's cost, the coordinated care program aims to reduce expenses for Stanford's self-funded insurance plan. The goal of this strategy is to empower individuals with chronic

illnesses to stay away from having repeated setbacks, reducing the likelihood of hospital readmissions and other complications. Everyone on the team has a good grasp of the patients and works to achieve the objectives that the patients themselves articulate.

24. Glaseroff states that the fundamental approach is to engage with people, simply sit and converse with them, and treat them with respect. The key to connecting with children, he adds, is listening and paying attention to their concerns, no matter how insignificant they may appear in comparison to our own. It is not, in my opinion, a minor matter. It ends up being really important.

25. Glaseroff maintains that the method can be successfully implemented in any field of medicine that exhibits continuity. "You can't expect to walk in, complete the task at hand, and then disappear," he explains.

26. "We discovered that patients would put extraordinary efforts if we trained everyone in this approach and were really consistent with it."

27. Zulman expresses that she is intrigued by the possibility of overcoming obstacles to such achievements by implementing something that appears "vast and fairly abstract" into practical interventions that benefit clinicians.

28. This might lead to new ways of obtaining patients' histories and doing exams that emphasize face-to-face interaction, or it could pave the way for more autonomy for doctors to spend more time with each patient and less time working with EHRs.

29. "To be honest, it's a very difficult problem," Zulman remarks. "If there were an easy way, and all you had to do was look me in the eye, we would have solved it long ago."

New Words and Expressions

New Words and
Expressions

oncology /ɒŋˈkɒlədʒi/ n. the scientific study of and treatment of tumors in the body 肿瘤学

pathology /pəˈθɒlədʒi/ n. the scientific study of diseases 病理学

undetected /ˌʌndɪˈtektɪd/ adj. not noticed by anyone 未被注意的

scour /ˈskaʊə(r)/ v. to search a place or thing thoroughly in order to find sb./sth. (彻底地)搜寻; 搜查; 翻找

death sentence the legal punishment of being killed for a serious crime 死刑

will /wɪl/ v. to use the power of your mind to do sth. or to make sth. happen 立定志向；决心；决意

matter-of-fact /ˌmætər əv ˈfækt/ adj. said or done without showing any emotion, especially in a situation in which you would expect sb. to express their feelings 不动感情的；据实的

chemotherapy /ˌkiːməʊˈθerəpi/ n. the treatment of disease, especially cancer, with the use of chemical substances(尤指对癌的)化学治疗；化学疗法；化疗

facade /fəˈsɑːd/ n. the way that sb./sth. appears to be, which is different from the way sb. / sth. really is(虚假的)表面；外表

ballgame /bɔlˈgeɪm/ n. a particular situation that is radically different from the preceding situation 情况；局面

poignant /ˈpɔɪnjənt/ adj. having a strong effect on your feelings, especially in a way that makes you feel sad 令人沉痛的；悲惨的；酸楚的

compassion /kəmˈpæʃn/ n. a strong feeling of sympathy for people who are suffering and a desire to help them 同情；怜悯

adjunct professor a part-time faculty member who teaches specific courses at a college or university but is not typically involved in the institution's administration, research, or other full-time faculty responsibilities 兼职教授；客座教授

glean /gliːn/ v. to obtain information, knowledge etc., sometimes with difficulty and often from various different places 费力地收集；四处搜集(信息、知识等)

setback /ˈsetbæk/ n. a difficulty or problem that delays or prevents sth., or makes a situation worse 挫折；阻碍

intrigue /ɪnˈtriːg/ v. to make sb. very interested and want to know more about sth. 激起……的兴趣；引发……的好奇心

implement /ˈɪmplɪmənt/ v. to make sth. that has been officially decided start to happen or be used 使生效；贯彻；执行；实施

intervention /ˌɪntəˈvenʃn/ n. care provided to improve a situation (especially medical procedures or applications that are intended to relieve illness or injury) 干预

clinician /klɪˈnɪʃn/ *n.* a doctor, psychologist, etc. who has direct contact with patients 临床医师

autonomy /ɔːˈtɒnəmi/ *n.* the ability to act and make decisions without being controlled by anyone else 自主；自主权

Notes

1. M.D.：doctor of medicine 医学博士

2. Alice in Wonderland：Alice is from *Alice's Adventures in Wonderland*, widely beloved British children's book by Lewis Carroll, published in 1865. With its fantastical tales and riddles, it became one of the most popular works of English-language fiction.

爱丽丝出自《爱丽丝梦游仙境》，这是刘易斯·卡罗尔于 1865 年出版的广受喜爱的英国儿童书籍。凭借其奇幻的故事和谜语，它成为了英语小说中最受欢迎的作品之一。

After Reading Activities

Reading Comprehension

Decide whether the following statements are true (T) or false (F) according to the text.

_____ 1. Kimberly Allison was diagnosed with breast cancer after she took the job at the University of Washington Medical Center's breast cancer pathology lab.

_____ 2. Allison tried to hide her feelings at the first meeting with her surgeon and two oncologists.

_____ 3. Kristine Calhoun gave Allision false hope that helped to keep her alive.

_____ 4. According to Lloyd Minor, the most a physician can do for suffering patients is to offer comfort by being an empathetic and understanding listener.

_____ 5. Alan Glaseroff pointed out that the way to engage with patients is listening, focusing on what they care about.

Words and Phrases

Match each English phrase in Column A with its Chinese version in Column B.

Column A	Column B
1. treatment plan	A. 肿瘤治疗团队
2. pathology lab	B. 病理学实验室
3. oncology team	C. 兼职教授
4. prognosis	D. 外科医生
5. adjunct professor	E. 内科医生
6. chronic illness	F. 慢性病
7. physician	G. 预后
8. surgeon	H. 治疗方案

Translation

我致力于改善床旁查体技能已达九年之久，这强调了在诊断过程中以及建立医患信任关系时个人互动的重要性。当一个实习生向我寻求关于病人的建议时，我的第一个回答是："我们现在不能作决定，我们需要先去看看病人。"你可以得到很多字里行间的信息——他们到底有多痛苦？他们真的不能呼吸吗？他们能用完整的句子和我说话吗？他们有多虚弱？我真的在努力了解这个人，那时，决策就会变得更好。

_____

_____

_____

_____

Critical Thinking

One factor that prevents doctors from spending time listening to patients is that most of them are suffering from burnout at work. Do you think this is true? What do you think we can do to help address the problem?

Part III   Apply Medical English

A. Situational Dialogues in Different Clinical Departments

Stomatology（口腔科）

Toothache（牙痛）

Dialogue

Doctor：Sorry to have kept you waiting. What can I do for you?

Patient：Doctor, I'm having trouble with a tooth in the upper left side. It has been hurting on and off for the past few weeks.

Doctor：Let me take a look to find out what's wrong. Please sit down in this chair. Open your mouth wide.

Patient：OK.

Doctor：There is a cavity in your tooth from the upper left side. And your gums are red and swollen.

Patient：Is it serious? The thought of tooth extraction makes me so anxious.

Doctor：That's completely understandable. Many people experience dental anxiety when they come to our office. But let me assure you that we are here to make your experience as pleasant as possible.

Patient：I really appreciate your help. Your words make me feel better.

Doctor：Don't worry too much. But we may take an X-ray just to be sure. We need to know your general health. Here are some standard medical questions. Please answer all the questions and take your time.

Patient：No problem.

Doctor：Well, the X-ray shows that you only have the adult gingivitis. And I can put filling in the cavity for you. You might feel a little bit uncomfortable but it won't hurt a lot.

Patient：OK. This is comforting.

Doctor：All right! We are finished. You will get better soon. And remember, it's essential to visit the dentist regularly for check-ups and cleanings to prevent any potential problems before they become severe. We want to keep your smile healthy and beautiful for years to come.

Patient：I see. Thank you very much!

🔲 Words and Phrases

cavity /ˈkævəti/ *n.* 蛀牙

gums /gʌmz/ *n.* 牙龈

tooth extraction /tuːθ ɪkˈstrækʃn/ 拔牙

dental anxiety /ˈdentl æŋˈzaɪəti/ 牙科治疗焦虑

appreciate /əˈpriːʃieɪt/ *v.* 感激

gingivitis /ˌdʒɪndʒɪˈvaɪtəs/ *n.* 牙龈炎

filling /ˈfɪlɪŋ/ *n.* 填充；填料

🔲 Notes

Stomatology is a branch of medicine that deals with the study, diagnosis, and treatment of diseases and conditions related to the mouth and jaw. It is a broader field than dentistry as it covers not only the teeth but also the gums, tongue, salivary glands, and other oral tissues.

Here are some most common diseases of stomatology.

Cavities

Cavities are one of the most common diseases people get and live with during their lifetime. Cavities are caused by the bacteria in your mouth that stick to your teeth. You feed the bacteria every time you eat or drink. The bacteria produce acid which starts to dissolve the outer enamel layer of your teeth. Your saliva clears away the acid and helps to repair the enamel. If the repair isn't fast enough, bacteria get inside your tooth and make cavities. Cavities will get bigger unless the bacteria are stopped or removed. You should visit your dentist regularly. Your dentist may recommend fluoride or other products to stop small cavities. You may need a filling to fix larger cavities. A tooth with a cavity near the nerve may need a root canal or to be pulled.

Gum disease

Gum disease refers to conditions that involve inflammation and infection of the tissues (gum and bone) that surround and support the teeth. Gum diseases, such as gingivitis and periodontitis, are largely preventable and treatable. The key is good oral hygiene, overall self-care, and regular care from a dental health care provider.

Cancers of the oral cavity and pharynx

Cancers of the oral cavity and pharynx include areas like the tongue, cheeks and gums, floor of the mouth, and the back of the throat. These cancers are primarily diagnosed in older adults, particularly those with a history of tobacco and alcohol use. A portion of these cancers may also be associated with infection with human papillomavirus (HPV). To help prevent cancers of the oral cavity and pharynx, limit alcohol and do not use tobacco. Speak to your doctor about HPV vaccination, which can prevent new infections of certain types of HPV that can cause oropharyngeal cancers.

　

口腔科是医学的一个分支,主要研究、诊断和治疗与口腔和颌骨有关的疾病和病症。与牙科相比,口腔科的范围更广,不仅包括牙齿,还包括牙龈、舌头、唾液腺和其他口腔组织。

以下是一些最常见的口腔疾病:

蛀牙

蛀牙是人们一生中最常见的疾病之一。蛀牙是由口腔中附着在牙齿上的细菌引起的。每次进食或饮水都会给细菌提供营养。细菌产生的酸会溶解牙齿的外层牙釉质。唾液可以清除酸性物质,帮助修复牙釉质。如果修复不够快,细菌会进入牙齿并形成蛀牙。除非细菌被阻止或清除,否则蛀牙会越来越大。人们应该定期去看牙医。牙医可能会推荐氟化物或其他产品来阻止小蛀洞扩大。较大的蛀洞可能需要填充物来修复。神经附近有蛀洞的牙齿可能需要进行根管治疗或被拔掉。

牙龈疾病

牙龈疾病是指周围和支持牙齿的组织(牙龈和骨骼)的炎症和感染。牙龈疾病,如牙龈炎和牙周炎,在很大程度上是可预防和治疗的。关键是良好的口腔卫生、全面的自我保健以及定期接受牙科保健服务。

口腔和咽部癌症

口腔和咽部癌症涉及的区域包括舌头、脸颊和牙龈、口底和喉咙后部等部位。这些癌症主要确诊于老年人,特别是有吸烟史和饮酒史的人。部分癌症还可能与人乳头状瘤病毒(HPV)感染有关。为帮助预防口腔和咽部癌症,应限制饮酒,不吸烟。同时也可以向医生咨询 HPV 疫苗接种事宜,这些疫苗可预防某些导致口腔和咽部癌症的 HPV 病毒感染。

Practical Activity

Work with your partner to create and perform a doctor-patient dialogue related to diseases of stomatology.

B. Practical Unit Project

Please write an essay on Practical Strategies for Better Doctor-Patient Communication with no less than 200 words.

Guidance for
Production

Tips for writing this essay:

1. Write an introduction.

Give a brief introduction of doctor-patient communication and demonstrate why it is a matter of concern.

2. Write the body part.

One paragraph only illustrates one idea which is stated clearly by a topic sentence.

- The entire discussion: the examples, details, and explanations in a particular paragraph must directly relate to and support the topic sentence.

- A good paragraph has unity. A paragraph must stick to its announced subject; it must not drift away into another discussion.

For example: You may write one paragraph to talk about what doctors can do concerning *verbal communication skills*, such as using clear, straightforward language suited to each patient's educational and cultural background, replacing medical jargon with more commonly used words, etc.. You may write another paragraph which focuses on *non-verbal communication skills*, such as listening attentively to the patient's words, showing support and concern by using appropriate gestures, offering written information to clarify the key medical information so as to avoid misunderstanding and so on.

Using transitional words and phrases. Transitional words and phrases help the reader move smoothly from one thought to the next so that the ideas do not appear disconnected or choppy.

Here is a list of common transitional words and phrases:

Giving examples: for example, for instance, specifically, in particular, namely, another, other, in addition, to illustrate;

Comparison: similarly, not only... but also..., in comparison;

Contrast: although, but, while, in contrast, however, though, on the other hand, nevertheless;

Sequence: first, second, third, finally, moreover, also, in addition, next, then, after, furthermore, and, previously;

Results: therefore, thus, consequently, as a result.

3. Write a conclusion.

The conclusion gives the reader a sense of completion on the subject and emphasizes the validity and importance of the topic.

Part IV   Self-Assessment

Use the following self-assessment checklist to check what you have learned in this unit.

I understand the impact of doctor-patient communication in health care.	☐
I can identify and use the words, phrases and sentence patterns related to the topic.	☐
I can write an essay by using the terminologies and medical information in this unit.	☐
I know the importance and skills of maintaining a good doctor-patient communication.	☐

Unit 7
Narrative Medicine

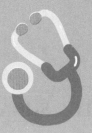

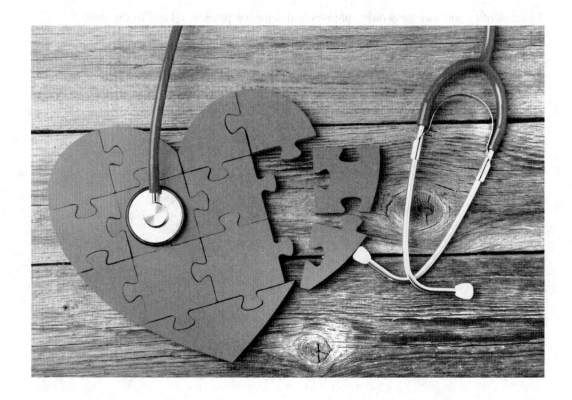

Narrative medicine is a medical approach that utilizes people's narratives in clinical practice, research, and education as a way to promote healing. It aims to address the relational and psychological dimensions, with an attempt to deal with the individual stories of patients. In doing this, narrative medicine aims not only to validate the experience of the patient, but also to encourage creativity and self-reflection in the physician.

Lead in

This unit is mainly to achieve the following objectives:

1) Understand the concept of narrative medicine;

2) Identify words, phrases and sentence patterns related to the topic;

3) Write a letter telling a doctor-patient story by using the terminologies and medical information in this unit;

4) Understand how narrative medicine affects doctor-patient relationship.

Part I　View the Medical World

Watch a video about narrative medicine and choose the right answer.①

1. Which of the following aspects is not included in the consideration of narrative medicine?

　　A. Physical.　　　　　　　　　　　B. Mental.

　　C. Rational.　　　　　　　　　　　D. Emotional.

2. Narrative medicine includes all of the following skills except _____.

　　A. the ability to listen　　　　　　C. the ability to comprehend

　　B. the ability to count　　　　　　D. the ability to act upon

3. Clinicians can gain _____ by seeking out a patient's story.

　　A. an in-depth perspective　　　　C. a yes or no answer

　　B. a once in a life time experience　D. a memorable experience

4. How many divides are there that hamper the development of a strong patient-clinician connection?

　　A. 1.　　　　　　　　　　　　　　B. 2.

　　C. 3.　　　　　　　　　　　　　　D. 4.

5. _____ makes the process of diagnosis and treatment more difficult and stressful.

　　A. Patients' hesitation to share personal details

　　B. Clinicians' strong willingness to inquire

　　C. Patients' cooperation

　　D. Clinicians' expertise

Words and Phrases

lay the foundation /leɪ ðə faʊnˈdeɪʃn/ 奠定基础

reflect /rɪˈflekt/ v. 显示；表明；表达

---

① 视频详见网站：https://pan-yz. cldisk. com/external/m/file/1055138655932473344。

critical /ˈkrɪtɪkl/ *adj.* 关键的

contextualize /kənˈtekstʃuəlaɪz/ *v.* 将……置于背景中考虑

an array of /ən əˈreɪ ɒv/ 一系列；大量的

nuance /ˈnjuːɑːns/ *n.* 细微差别

invalidate /ɪnˈvælɪdeɪt/ *v.* 证明……错误；使站不住脚

marginalized /ˈmɑːdʒɪnəlaɪzd/ *v.* 使处于边缘

categorical trauma /ˌkætəˈɡɒrɪkl ˈtrɔːmə/ 范畴性创伤

divide /dɪˈvaɪd/ *n.* 差异；分歧

hamper /ˈhæmpə(r)/ *v.* 阻碍；妨碍

vulnerability /ˌvʌlnərəˈbɪlətɪ/ *n.* 脆弱性

Part II   Read to Explore Medical Knowledge

Text A

Pre-reading Questions:

1. Have you ever heard of the term Narrative Medicine?

2. What happens when doctors fail to recognize the importance of listening and how can they cope with this problem?

Narrative Medicine in Medical Diagnosis

Text A

1. In the medical area, patients' quality of life and the accuracy of disease diagnoses have both been enhanced by the scientific breakthroughs brought about by modernity. Nobody can deny this. All it takes is a little creative thinking to switch our lives to two distinct periods in history: the Renaissance and the modern day. Leaving cultural or historical affinities aside, which one of these would you most prefer to live in? The present century is probably the best time to respond prudently. There is a long line of thinkers who contributed to medical progress—names like Vesalius and Paré come to mind—but it is undeniable that the 20th century was a watershed moment in medical history.

2. The greatest scientific discoveries in every discipline have been achieved in the last hundred years, yet modernism has also altered the nature of time. The creation of goods and information, the development of interpersonal relationships, and the rate of communication unfold at rates that were previously inconceivable. It is important to emphasize the latter point and timely mention the changes that have occurred as a result of the intensification of the relationship between doctors and their patients. Life seems to be meant to be mechanically produced in accordance with Fordist logic. There are a number of areas that

have been significantly expedited, including the development of new diagnostic tests, surgeries, and medications, as well as the rapid response to medical emergencies. However, it appears that all aspects of life, including what must inevitably be put on hold, are being swept along by these benefits. "Produce more and more in less time" appears to be the mantra. Being "better" requires us to be productive.

3. There is no longer any doubt that health staff, and doctors in particular, have given up their practice to this phrase. Whether operating under a public or private guise, health care organizations act in a utilitarian manner. Gains in "better" statistics or income are the end result of their pursuit of maximum returns. The service time is becoming shorter due to the necessity of attending to a specific number of patients per hour. The patient is not thoroughly evaluated, and in exchange, a battery of imaging and laboratory testing is sought in order to arrive at a diagnosis. This is obviously not new to the people who do it for a living; after all, it is a core component of medical education to focus on the outward manifestations of disease. Strategies for gaining access to the patient's experience and inner world receive almost minimal attention. Storytelling opportunities like the one highlighted by Paco Maglio do arise from time to time: I was once requested to take the pulse of an elderly woman (the diminutive is really kind). Without agreeing to her request, I looked at the cardioscope and reassured her, "Don't worry, Grandma. You are 80 years old, and you are doing very well." Nevertheless, she persisted in having me take her pulse, and at her insistence I questioned her why, given how consistently accurate the machine was. She finally spoke up: "It is that nobody touches me here." While we did not physically touch her, we did palpate her.

4. What does this finding suggest? That maybe the doctor-patient interaction has lost something crucial. Acting with a strong technical vision, i. e., applying one's knowledge and abilities to cure the patient, is commonplace in the health care industry. This is done well and morally, but it has been overlooked that a patient is more than just corporality; in such cases, one must take on the role of a doctor, combining healing skills with a loving attitude. The use of the cardioscope and physical contact with the patient are both crucial. That being said, "doctor: good person, full of humanity, proficient in the art of healing" is an old Latin adage that serves as a moral code for medical professionals.

5. Narrative medicine was established to return to a fuller picture of the patient. Dr. Rita

Charon came up with this word, and it's meant to provide an alternative perspective to present orthodoxy. Two steps comprise this narrative practice: first, a medical practice that is imbued with storytelling abilities that enable doctors to hear, understand, and be moved by patients' stories—all while maintaining a framework of respect for the individual impacted by the illness—and second, the cultivation of medical professionals through the experiences gained from this approach to the patient.

6. In most circumstances, this will need doctors to be humble and to adopt a new position, away from "their seat" or "pedestal" where they hold power. The domains of the incommunicable or extremely difficult to communicate cannot be entered by doctors unless they join their patients on their journeys, are constantly moving around with them, and find a vibrant, precise, and metaphorical language to describe what appears to be incommunicable, according to Oliver Sacks.

7. Put another way, trying to find a language that both parties can understand means bridging the gap between doctors and patients, sometimes swimming together and other times falling into the abyss that separates them. Being a patient doesn't imply appropriating their pain— that would drastically reduce medical intervention—but rather, it means getting to know them. You can't reach a place of empathy unless you lower the shield.

8. Through sympathy or empathy, doctors should advance in the company of patients, sharing their experiences, thoughts, and feelings—that is, the intimate concepts that comprise their behavior—rather than viewing patients as impersonal objects, identifying themselves with them, or turning it into a projection of themselves. They need to be able to put themselves in their patients' shoes without letting it affect them, and they should also strive to help their patients do the same by juggling two sets of priorities simultaneously.

9. The goal of using the narrative style in medical education is to bring that relegated language back. The doctor-patient relationship has been strengthened, clinical analysis of the cases studied has improved, and our understanding of disease diagnosis, prognosis, and therapy has deepened as a result of this technique. Furthermore, it can enhance the patient's involvement in shared decision-making processes. Since the official medical history and the narrative medicine are not antagonistic but rather complimentary, it is worthwhile to use the latter as a complement in addition to the former.

New Words and Expressions

affinity /əˈfɪnəti/ *n.* a close relationship between two people or things that have similar qualities, structures or features 密切的关系

prudently /ˈpruːdntli/ *adv.* sensible and careful when you make judgements and decisions; avoiding unnecessary risks 谨慎地;审慎地

unfold /ʌnˈfəʊld/ *v.* to spread open or flat sth. that has previously been folded; to become open and flat (使)展开;打开

medication /ˌmedɪˈkeɪʃn/ *n.* a drug or another form of medicine that you take to prevent or to treat an illness 药;药物

utilitarian /ˌjuːtɪlɪˈteəriən/ *adj.* designed to be useful and practical rather than attractive 实用的;功利的;实惠的

diminutive /dɪˈmɪnjətɪv/ *adj.* very small 微小的;极小的;特小的

cardioscope /ˈkɑːdiə(ʊ)skəʊp/ *n.* any of various instruments used to assess, inspect, or display information about the heart 心脏示波器;心脏镜;心电图示波器

insistence /ɪnˈsɪstəns/ *n.* an act of demanding or saying sth. firmly and refusing to accept any opposition or excuses 坚决要求;坚持;固执

palpate /pælˈpeɪt/ *v.* to examine part of the body by touching it 触诊;触摸检查

corporality /kɔːpəˈræliti/ *n.* the quality of being physical 肉体

orthodoxy /ˈɔːθədɒksi/ *n.* an idea or view that is generally accepted 普遍接受的观点

imbue /ɪmˈbjuː/ *v.* to fill sb./sth. with strong feelings, opinions or values 使充满;灌输;激发(强烈感情、想法或价值)

pedestal /ˈpedɪstl/ *n.* the base that a column, statue, etc. rests on (柱子或雕塑等的)底座;基座

domain /dəˈmeɪn/ *n.* an area of knowledge or activity; especially one that sb. is responsible for (知识、活动的)领域;范围;范畴

abyss /əˈbɪs/ *n.* a very deep wide space or hole that seems to have no bottom 深渊

appropriate /əˈprəʊpriət/ *v.* to take sth./sb.'s ideas, etc. for your own use, especially illegally or without permission 盗用;挪用;占用;侵吞

impersonal /ɪmˈpɜːsənl/ *adj.* lacking friendly human feelings or atmosphere; making you feel unimportant 缺乏人情味的；冷淡的

projection /prəˈdʒekʃn/ *n.* the act of putting an image of sth. onto a surface; an image that is shown in this way 投射；放映；投影；放映的影像

simultaneously /ˌsɪmlˈteɪniəslɪ/ *adv.* happening or done at the same time as sth. else 同时发生(或进行)地；同步地

relegate /ˈrelɪɡeɪt/ *v.* to give sb. a lower or less important position, rank, etc. than before 使贬职；使降级；降低……的地位

prognosis /prɒɡˈnəʊsɪs/ *n.* an opinion, based on medical experience, of the likely development of a disease or an illness (对病情的)预断；预后

antagonistic /ænˌtæɡəˈnɪstɪk/ *adj.* showing or feeling opposition 敌对的；敌意的

complement /ˈkɒmplɪmənt/ *v.* add to sth. in a way that improves it or makes it more attractive 补充；补足；使完美；使更具吸引力

🗒 Notes

1. Renaissance：It refers to the humanistic revival of classical art, architecture, literature, and learning that originated in Italy in the 14th century and later spread throughout Europe. The period of this revival, roughly went through from the 14th to the 16th century, marking the transition from medieval to modern times.

文艺复兴指的是古典艺术、建筑、文学和学术的人文主义复兴，起源于 14 世纪的意大利，后来传播到整个欧洲。这一复兴时期大致是从 14 世纪到 16 世纪，标志着从中世纪向现代的过渡。

2. Andreas Vesalius（1514-1564）：He was an anatomist and physician who wrote *De Humani Corporis Fabrica Libri Septem* (*On the fabric of the human body in seven books*), what is considered to be one of the most influential books on human anatomy. Vesalius is often referred to as the founder of modern human anatomy.

安德烈亚斯·维萨留斯(1514—1564)是一位解剖学家和医生，他撰写了《人体的构造》(七卷本)，该书被认为是最有影响力的人类解剖学著作之一。维萨留斯常被誉为现代

人体解剖学的创始人。

3. Ambroise Paré（1510-1590）: He was a French surgeon who served in that role for kings Henry II, Francois II, Charles IX and Henry III. He is considered one of the fathers of surgery and modern forensic pathology and a pioneer in surgical techniques and battlefield medicine, especially in the treatment of wounds. He was also an anatomist, invented several surgical instruments, and was a member of the Parisian surgeon guild.

安布鲁瓦·帕雷（1510—1590）是一位法国外科医生，曾为亨利二世、弗朗索瓦二世、查理九世和亨利三世等国王服务。他被认为是现代外科学和法医学的奠基人之一，也是外科技术和战地医学的先驱，特别是在伤口治疗方面。他还是一位解剖学家，发明了几种外科手术器械，并且是巴黎外科行会的成员。

4. Fordist Logic: It has something to do with Fordism, the theory of Henry Ford, for which he states that production efficiency is dependent on successful assembly-line methods.

福特主义逻辑与亨利·福特的理论"福特主义"有关，福特认为生产效率的提高取决于成功的流水线作业方法。

5. Rita Charon: Rita Charon is a prominent figure in the field of narrative medicine. She is a physician, educator, and writer, widely recognized as the originator of the concept of narrative medicine. She holds an M. D. degree and a PhD in English, which reflects her interdisciplinary approach to health care and literature.

丽塔·卡伦是叙事医学领域的杰出人物。她是一位医生、教育家和作家，被普遍认为是叙事医学概念的鼻祖。她同时拥有医学博士学位和英语博士学位，这使得她能运用针对医疗保健和文学领域的跨学科研究方法。

After Reading Activities

Reading Comprehension

I. Answer the following questions.

1. According to the author, when is the most favorable era for people to live in and why?

2. How does the Fordist Logic affect people's ways of living?

3. What are the two movements involved in the narrative practice?

4. Describe your understanding of "the incommunicable". What could "the incommunicable" be?

5. How can the techniques of narrative medicine help treat patients in the medical field?

✅ II. Work in groups to complete the following chart according to the structure of the text.

Modernity is a double-edged sword. (paras. 1-2)

1. Modernity has brought great _____. Given the choices of living either in _____ or _____, the answer is self-evident, because the history of medicine experienced _____ in the 20th century. (para. 1)

2. Due to the unprecedentedly fast development of technology, many things such as _____ , _____ and _____ have been changed. But the intensification of the _____ is worth our attention. (para. 2)

Problems occur when doctors ignore patients' experience and internal world. (paras. 3-5)

1. To have maximum returns, namely "better" _____ or _____, health personnel or doctors pay little attention to _____. (para. 3)

2. Something crucial is missing in the _____. Therefore, a doctor must combine _____ with _____. (para. 4)

3. Narrative medicine works by first, a medical practice _____ and second, _____ through the experiences resulting from this approach to the patient. (para. 5)

What can doctors do to cope with the problem? (paras. 6-8)

1. Doctors need to step down from "their seat" or _____. (para. 6)

2. Doctors need to look for a _____. (para. 7)

3. Doctors should not see patients as _____. (para. 8)

Conclusion: the advantages of using the narrative techniques in the field of medical education (para. 9)

The strategy has shown positive results. And it is worth _____ as a complement to the official medical history.

Words and Phrases

✅ I. Translate the following medical terms into Chinese or English.

1. narrative medicine   _____

2. doctor-patient relationship   _____

3. improve the clinical analysis   _____

4. moral code   _____

5. 对紧急事件的快速反应   _____

6. 疾病的诊断和治疗   _____

7. 培养医学专业人才   _____

8. 医疗干预   _____

✅ II. Fill in the blanks with the words or phrases given below. Change the form if necessary.

insistence on	unfold	prudent	medication	antagonistic

1. He quickly _____ the blankets and spread them on the mattress.

2. He admired your _____ understanding things and making your point, even when he preferred his own.

3. Each couple of the research traditions is incommensurable and mutually complemental, but not opposite and _____ .

4. It might be more _____ to get a second opinion before going ahead.

5. Many flu _____ are available without a prescription.

Sentence Translation

Translate the following sentences into Chinese or English.

1. The domains of the incommunicable or extremely difficult to communicate cannot be entered by doctors unless they join their patients on their journeys, which are constantly moving

around with them, and find a vibrant, precise, and metaphorical language to describe what appears to be incommunicable.

_____

_____

2. Two steps comprise this narrative practice: first, a medical practice that is imbued with storytelling abilities that enable doctors to hear, understand, and be moved by patients' stories—all while maintaining a framework of respect for the individual impacted by the illness—and second, the cultivation of medical professionals through the experiences gained from this approach to the patient.

_____

_____

3. The creation of goods and information, the development of interpersonal relationships, and the rate of communication unfold at rates that were previously inconceivable.

_____

_____

4. 为了对患者有更全面的了解，叙事医学应运而生。这个词是由丽塔·卡伦(Rita Charon)博士创造的，意在为目前的正统观念提供另一种视角。

_____

_____

5. 由于每小时必须接待特定数量的病人，服务时间越来越短。病人没有得到彻底的评估，换来的是一系列影像和实验室检查，以得出诊断结果。

_____

_____

Text B

Pre-reading Questions:

1. What is the significance of recognizing that every patient has a story that goes beyond their symptoms?

2. How can stories of patients illuminate their illness and the social challenges they face during recovery?

Narrative Medicine: The Unique Story of Each Patient

Text B

1. There is more to every patient's narrative than just the symptoms they present with when they visit the doctor. These accounts can illuminate individual's journey to health, the moment of crisis that compelled them to reach out for assistance, and most significantly, the societal obstacles they encounter while they recover. By providing the kind of contextual richness that nourishes empathy, stories might encourage health care providers to shift their focus from "How can I cure this disease?" to "How can I assist my patient?" Supporters of what is referred to as "narrative medicine" argue that understanding how to encourage patients to tell their stories can have a transformative impact on the quality of patient treatment, even though the approach may appear insignificant at first.

2. That kind of epiphany came to Indu Voruganti, MS, a third-year medical student at Brown University's Warren Alpert Medical School. After finishing her bachelor's degree in biology, Voruganti's original aim was to instantly enroll in medical school. Nonetheless, she chose to take a slight detour a little after enrolling in an undergraduate creative writing class.

3. Voruganti stated, "I immediately felt creative writing exercised a unique part of my brain that seemed to offer a different lens with which to view health care." I discovered that there is a vast community of doctors who also write when that happened.

4. Voruganti enrolled in the interdisciplinary master's program at Columbia University College of Physicians and Surgeons called the Program in Narrative Medicine after having that "aha！" moment. The program's goal is to enhance clinical care by means of narratives. Simply put, narrative medicine encourages students to broaden their understanding of patients beyond their medical history through the study of art and literature, which in turn improves their listening and observational skills.

5. Voruganti, who in 2015 developed and taught an elective course on Art and the Narrative Medicine to first- and second-year Brown medical students, stated, "Narrative medicine can help us deliver more humanistic health care."

Amassing the Skill of Empathy

6. The area of narrative medicine was founded by Rita Charon, M.D., PhD, who is also the executive director of Columbia's Program in Narrative Medicine. In a paper published in 2001 in *JAMA*, Charon argued that being able to "acknowledge, absorb, interpret, and act on the stories and plights of others" is essential for successful medical practice.

7. "It's clear that we require assistance in analyzing our own procedures and comprehending and valuing the feedback we receive from patients. After Charon began using narrative skills in her professional work, she realized that it may help her patients feel better heard and valued. It's a promise to learn about patients' experiences, support those who care for them, and speak up for those who are suffering.

8. Learning to close "read," or examine a text with care and analysis, is an essential part of narrative medicine course work. Through this method, students can learn empathetic listening skills which will help them connect with patients on a deeper level. These days, first-year medical students at Columbia University are required to take one of fourteen seminars including narrative medicine, visual arts, medical journalism, and memoir writing. Under Charon's direction, the medical school also provides a scholarly track in Narrative and Social Medicine and a fourth-year elective for medical students.

9. Numerous medical institutions have incorporated narrative medicine into their curricula, with Columbia University being the sole institution to grant a master degree in the field. Medical students at UNR's School of Medicine have the option to take narrative medicine

either as a fourth-year elective or as a scholarly specialization. Students are required to write and submit a reflective essay of 10,000 words on clinical experiences to a medical humanities journal as part of their course work. Although many students dabble in fiction and poetry, narrative medicine professor Susan Palwick (PhD) at UNR has found that most students are primarily interested in writing personal essays.

10. It's easy to reduce persons to a single ailment, according to Palwick, an associate professor in the Office of Medical Education at UNR and an associate professor of English. As a method of maintaining an inquisitive attitude toward patients, narrative medicine helps put pieces back together. In the end, it's just love.

11. She also mentioned that students can learn to recognize and overcome their own biases through this experience. For example, according to Palwick, one student who felt especially critical of bariatric surgery patients decided to pen a collection of short stories exploring the mental health issues that make these people unable to reduce weight through more conventional means. "Helps you stay empathetic and sympathetic," Palwick found out about the process.

12. Reflective writing offers a "safe space" where students can openly address the challenges of medical school and their worries related to the profession, she further stated.

13. Fourth-year UNR medical student Jake Measom remarked that the narrative medicine academic specialization encouraged him to think outside the box when caring for patients. In addition, he considers narrative medicine a "remedy to burnout," saying that although being a doctor can seem boring at times, it helps him remember that "there's a story to be had everywhere."

14. "It not only improves my listening skills and compassionate feelings, but it also helps you understand yourself better," he said, adding, "It also makes me a better physician."

Relying on Narratives for Emotional Support

15. "As long as you retrieve it, I will not worry if you cannot recall its exact location. Someone needs to rush to the basement and retrieve fresh scrubs for you if there is a significant amount of blood. Donning your coat, you enter the restroom. If you want to say it aloud, just look in the mirror. You refer to the mother by her maiden name and the child

by her given name. This part cannot be changed in any way."

16. This is a passage from an opinion article titled "How to Tell a Mother Her Child Is Dead," which was published in the September edition of the *New York Times* Sunday Review section last year. Authored by Naomi Rosenberg, M.D., a medical professional at Temple University Hospital, the piece serves as a heart-wrenching depiction of how narrative medicine can assist physicians in coping with the harrowing experiences they encounter on a daily basis.

17. In his new position as director of narrative medicine at Temple University Lewis Katz School of Medicine, Pulitzer Prize-winning writer Michael Vitez pushed Rosenberg to submit the story. Following a 30-year tenure as a journalist for the Philadelphia Inquirer, Vitez approached the dean of the school with the idea of utilizing his expertise to assist students, teachers, and patients in putting their experiences into words. In 2016, the concept morphed into Temple University's new Narrative Medicine Program.

18. With teachers and students working one-on-one with Vitez on their story works, the Temple program is now rather unstructured. "It helped her process her emotions and turn a really bad day into something really valuable," Vitez observed of a third-year medical student who recently sent him a poem she had written following a particularly trying day during her psychiatric rotation. A master's degree and certificate in narrative medicine are on the horizon at Temple.

19. "I believe that stories have an incredible power." Vitez stated, "Connecting with your patients, understanding them, and building relationships with them can be achieved by learning how to interview and ask questions and by understanding the value of a good story."

20. The narrative medicine course at Brown University's Warren Alpert Medical School, which is led by associate professor of emergency medicine Jay Baruch, M.D., also believes that medical schools should prioritize teaching students to think creatively, the kind of thinking that is typically associated with the humanities and the arts. " The anatomy of a patient's story just as much as the anatomy of the human body," he stated, emphasizing the importance of this knowledge for both students and clinicians.

New Words and Expressions

illuminate /ɪˈluːmɪneɪt/ *v.* to light up or make something clearer by shining light on it, or to explain and make something easier to understand 阐明；启发

compel /kəmˈpel/ *v.* to force or strongly persuade someone to do something 强迫；驱使

contextual /kənˈtekstʃuəl/ *n.* the depth and complexity added to something by its context, providing a deeper understanding 上下文的；与语境相关的

nourish /ˈnʌrɪʃ/ *v.* to provide with the substances necessary for growth, health, and good condition 滋养；养育

empathy /ˈempəθi/ *n.* the ability to understand and share the feelings of another person 共情；同感

provider /prəˈvaɪdər/ *n.* a person or organization that supplies goods or services 供应商；提供者

transformative /trænsˈfɔːmətɪv/ *adj.* causing a marked change or transformation 变革性的

approach /əˈprəʊtʃ/ *n.* a way of dealing with something 方法；途径

enroll /ɪnˈrəʊl/ *v.* to officially register as a member of an institution or a course of study 注册；加入

detour /ˈdiːtʊər/ *n.* a long or roundabout route taken to avoid something or to visit somewhere along the way 绕行；弯路

interdisciplinary /ˌɪntədɪsəˈplɪnəri/ *adj.* involving two or more academic disciplines or fields of study 跨学科的

acknowledge /əkˈnɒlɪdʒ/ *v.* to recognize or admit the existence, truth, or fact of something 承认；确认

absorb /əbˈzɔːb/ *v.* to take in or soak up a liquid or other substance; to understand and learn something thoroughly 吸收；领会

interpret /ɪnˈtɜːprət/ *v.* to explain the meaning of something; to understand something in a particular way 解释；理解

plight /plaɪt/ *n.* a difficult or distressing situation 困境；苦境

empathetic /ˌempəˈθetɪk/ *adj*. having the ability to understand and share the feelings of another person, showing empathy 善解人意的

seminar /ˈsemɪnɑː(r)/ *n*. any meeting for an exchange of ideas; or a course offered for a small group of advanced students 研讨会；讲座

compassionate /kəmˈpæʃənət/ *adj*. feeling or showing sympathy and concern for others, especially those who are suffering 富有同情心的；怜悯的

heart-wrenching /ˈhɑːt ˌrentʃɪŋ/ *adj*. causing intense sadness or distress; emotionally painful 令人心碎的；令人痛苦的

harrowing /ˈhærəʊɪŋ/ *adj*. extremely distressing or disturbing; causing feelings of fear or horror 令人痛苦的；令人恐惧的

morph /mɔːf/ *v*. to undergo a gradual and usually complete change of form, structure, or substance 逐渐变形；转变

rotation /rəʊˈteɪʃn/ *n*. the act of turning around a central point or axis; a regular cycle 轮换；旋转

emergency /ɪˈmɜːdʒənsi/ *n*. a serious, unexpected, and often dangerous situation requiring immediate action 紧急情况；突发事件

anatomy /əˈnætəmi/ *n*. the scientific study of the structure of living things, especially the body 解剖学

🔲 Notes

1. Program in Narrative Medicine: The Program in Narrative Medicine at Columbia University College of Physicians and Surgeons is an interdisciplinary initiative that integrates the art of storytelling and narrative skills into the practice of medicine and health care education. Founded by Dr. Rita Charon, the program aims to foster a deeper understanding of patients' experiences, enhance communication between health care professionals and patients, and promote empathy and humanism in medical care.

哥伦比亚大学内外科医学院的叙事医学项目是一个跨学科的项目，将讲故事的艺术

和叙事技巧融入医学和医疗保健教育的实践。该项目由丽塔·卡伦博士创立，旨在加深对患者经历的理解，加强医护人员与患者之间的沟通，增强医疗中的同理心和人道主义。

2. Michael Vitez：Michael Vitez is a Pulitzer Prize-winning journalist and educator known for his involvement in narrative medicine. He is recognized for his contributions to the field by using storytelling to bridge the gap between medical professionals, patients, and the public. Vitez's work highlights the power of narratives in conveying the emotional and personal aspects of health care experiences.

迈克尔·维特斯是普利策奖获奖记者和教育家，因其对叙事医学的研究而闻名。他通过讲故事的方式来弥合医疗专业人员、患者和公众之间的鸿沟。他因其对该领域的贡献而广受认可。迈克尔·维特斯的作品强调了叙事在传达医疗体验的情感和个人方面的重要作用。

📄 After Reading Activities

Reading Comprehension

Decide whether the following statements are true (T) or false (F) according to the text.

_____ 1. Narrative medicine seeks to enhance clinical care through the study of literature and art to improve students' listening and observation skills.

_____ 2. Indu Voruganti decided to enroll in the Program in Narrative Medicine at Columbia University after completing her medical studies.

_____ 3. The development of narrative competence benefits patients, not health care providers.

_____ 4. Students at the University of Nevada, Reno (UNR) School of Medicine are required to write personal essays for their narrative medicine assignments.

_____ 5. Narrative medicine can help students challenge their biases and develop curiosity about patients' experiences.

Words and Phrases

Match each English phrase in Column A with its Chinese version in Column B.

Column A	Column B
1. emergency medicine	A. 医学新闻
2. visual arts	B. 轮班轮岗
3. medical journalism	C. 视觉艺术
4. reflective writing	D. 急诊医学
5. humanistic health care	E. 跨学科的
6. empathetic listening	F. 共情倾听
7. interdisciplinary	G. 反思性写作
8. rotation	H. 人文医疗

Translation

　　叙事医学是一种医疗实践和教育方法，旨在通过借鉴文学和叙事的技巧，提高医务人员对患者的人文关怀、同理心和医学思考的能力。它强调医务人员不仅应该关注患者的身体症状和病史，还应该理解他们的个人故事、背景和情感体验，从而更全面地了解患者的需求和关切。医学叙事文本弥合了医学术语和人类情感之间的鸿沟，让患者分享他们的经验，让医护人员倾听和理解。

Critical Thinking

　　How does the incorporation of narrative medicine techniques in medical practice enhance communication between health care providers and patients? Conduct a study to assess, and collect qualitative data through interviews and surveys to gauge patients' perceptions of improved interactions and understanding.

Part III Apply Medical English

✅ A. Situational Dialogues in Different Clinical Departments

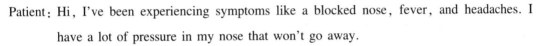

Dialogue

Otolaryngology（耳鼻喉科）

Sinusitis（鼻窦炎）

Doctor：Good morning, how can I help you today?

Patient：Hi, I've been experiencing symptoms like a blocked nose, fever, and headaches. I have a lot of pressure in my nose that won't go away.

Doctor：Have you noticed any changes in your breathing or voice?

Patient：My breathing has been a bit congested, and my voice sounds hoarse.

Doctor：These symptoms sound like they could be related to sinusitis. Have you had any other health issues recently?

Patient：No, I haven't had any major health problems recently. Just the occasional cold or sore throat.

Doctor：Let me take a listen. (*The doctor performs a physical exam and listens to the patient's lungs and heart with a stethoscope.*) Based on what I'm hearing, it seems like you have a mild case of sinusitis.

Patient：What should I do? Is there anything I can take for relief?

Doctor：You can try over-the-counter pain relievers like acetaminophen or ibuprofen to help with the pain and fever. You can also use a humidifier or saline spray to help relieve congestion. However, if your symptoms persist or worsen, you may need prescription medication or further treatment.

Patient：That sounds manageable.

Doctor：If your symptoms persist for more than a week or are severe, it might be best to see a neurologist or an allergist who can recommend additional tests or treatments. In the meantime, try to rest and avoid activities that trigger your symptoms.

Patient：Thank you for your advice. How long will it take for me to recover?

Doctor：Most cases of sinusitis resolve within a few weeks with home care and over-the-

205

counter medications. However, some people may experience chronic sinusitis that requires ongoing treatment. It's important to follow up with your primary care provider if your symptoms don't improve or become severe.

📋 Words and Phrases

congested /kən'dʒestɪd/ *adj.* 堵塞的

sinusitis /ˌsaɪnə'saɪtɪs/ *n.* 鼻窦炎

over-the-counter /ˌəʊvə ðə 'kaʊntə(r)/ *adj.* 非处方的

pain reliever /peɪn rɪ'liːvə(r)/ 止疼药

acetaminophen /əˌsiːtə'mɪnəfen/ *n.* 对乙酰氨基酚

ibuprofen /ˌaɪbjuː'prəʊfen/ *n.* 布洛芬

humidifier /hjuː'mɪdɪfaɪə(r)/ *n.* 湿度调节器

saline spray /'seɪlaɪn spreɪ/ 盐水喷雾剂

neurologist /njʊə'rɒlədʒɪst/ *n.* 神经科医生

allergist /'ælədʒɪst/ *n.* 过敏症专科医生

📋 Notes

Otolaryngology is a medical speciality which is focused on the ears, nose, and throat. It is also called otolaryngology-head and neck surgery because specialists are trained in both medicine and surgery. An otolaryngologist is often called an ear, nose, and throat doctor, or an ENT for short. This medical specialty dates back to the 19th century, when doctors recognized that the head and neck contained a series of interconnected systems. Doctors developed techniques and tools for examining and treating problems of the head and neck, eventually forming a medical specialty.

Here are some most common diseases of otolaryngology.

Ear infections

Ear infections are one of the most prevalent ENT disorders. They occur when germs become trapped inside the middle ear. The eustachian tube, a tiny canal that originates in the ear and drains into the back of the throat, usually keeps unwanted germs out. If this tube is too small or becomes swollen shut by swelling or clogged by fluid and mucus, bacteria, or other microbes can enter the ear and cause an infection.

Strep throat

Strep is an abbreviation for a family of bacteria called Streptococci. Strep throat occurs when the throat and surrounding structures become infected with this germ. Notably absent in strep throat are a runny nose and cough. You may also suspect strep throat if you have been exposed to someone with a strep infection in the last two weeks. Children between the ages of 5 and 15 are most at risk. You are also more likely to get a strep infection during the winter months.

Sinusitis

Sinusitis occurs when a germ multiplies in the hollow recesses of the skull that surrounds your eyes and nose. The infection can become trapped, causing inflammation, pressure, and pain. Acute sinusitis is often secondary to a common cold, so you are more likely to get sinusitis during the winter months. Chronic sinusitis in which symptoms persist for more than 12 weeks may occur as a result of an untreated allergy or a chronic condition such as bronchial asthma.

Sleep apnea

Apnea is a medical term meaning to stop breathing. Sleep apnea is a disorder causing one to stop breathing for brief periods of time while sleeping. Many individuals with sleep apnea have been told by a spouse or family member that they snore, gasp, choke, or even stop breathing momentarily while sleeping. You are more likely to have sleep apnea if you are overweight, have enlarged tonsils, or take sedatives at bedtime.

耳鼻喉科是一门专注于耳、鼻、喉的医学专业。它也被称为"耳鼻咽喉头颈外科",因为医生们接受过医学和外科方面的培训。耳鼻喉科医生通常被简称为耳鼻喉医生,或耳鼻喉医师。这一医学专科可追溯到19世纪,当时医生们认识到头颈部包含一系列相互联系的系统。医生们开发了检查和治疗头颈部问题的技术和工具,最终形成了一个医学专科。

以下是耳鼻喉科最常见的几种疾病。

中耳炎

中耳炎是耳鼻喉科最常见的疾病之一。当病菌被困在中耳内时就会产生中耳炎。咽鼓管是一条发源于耳朵并通向咽喉后部的细小管道，通常可以将有害病菌阻挡在外。如果咽鼓管太小或因肿胀而闭合，或被液体和黏液堵塞，细菌或其他微生物就会进入耳朵并引起感染。

链球菌性咽喉炎

Strep 是链球菌科细菌的缩写。当喉咙和周围组织感染这种病菌时，就会出现链球菌性咽喉炎。链球菌性咽喉炎主要表现为流鼻涕和咳嗽。如果您在过去两周内接触过链球菌感染者，您也有可能患上了链球菌性咽喉炎。5 至 15 岁的儿童为易感染人群。冬季发病率更高。

鼻窦炎

当病菌在眼鼻周围的颅骨内空腔繁殖时，就会引发鼻窦炎。感染分泌物不能及时排除可引起炎症、压迫和疼痛。急性鼻窦炎通常继发于普通感冒，因此在冬季更容易患上鼻窦炎。症状持续 12 周以上的鼻窦炎即为慢性鼻窦炎，病因可能是过敏或支气管哮喘等慢性疾病未得到治疗。

睡眠呼吸暂停

呼吸暂停是一个医学术语，意为呼吸停止。睡眠呼吸暂停是一种导致睡眠时短暂停止呼吸的疾病。许多患有睡眠呼吸暂停的人都曾被配偶或家人告知，他们在睡觉时会打鼾、喘气、窒息，甚至呼吸短时间停止。体重超重、扁桃体肥大或睡前服用镇静剂的人更容易患睡眠呼吸暂停。

▥ Practical Activity

Work with your partner to create and perform a doctor-patient dialogue related to diseases of otolaryngology.

✔ B. Practical Unit Project

Guidance for
Production

Please write a letter to one of your classmates, telling one doctor-patient story you knew or experienced during the internship with no less than 200 words.

Tips for writing this letter：

1. Brainstorm your ideas.

How do you like your internship experience in real medical practice? How is it different from your expectations? Do you encounter anyone special? What do you learn from people around you? You may try to recall what you heard, what you saw and how you and other people felt in a specific situation.

2. Work out an outline based on your ideas.

You may start your letter by telling your friend some basic information about your internship at a hospital including the time, the place, what you are supposed to do in the workplace, etc.. Then, you can tell the doctor-patient story in detail. There are several options of plotting the story. You can present the story in a chronological order, which means you can tell the story in time sequence. But you can also choose to intertwine some flashbacks within your story-telling, which might work better to impress your friend. At last, you may try to conclude your letter by talking about your feelings and what you have learned from the story.

3. Write and revise your letter.

While writing, it is better to select one episode and flesh it out with many specific details so that your friend can clearly see your point. Don't select a series of events whose retelling will be too long or complex for one theme. Also, you can present the story in a vivid way and provoke deeper thoughts by adopting sensory details such as the doctor's feeling on touching the skinny hands of the patient or using dialogues to imply the personalities of people. Remember to check your spellings and grammar when you finish the first draft.

Part IV   Self-Assessment

Use the following self-assessment checklist to check what you have learned in this unit.

I understand the concept of narrative medicine.	☐
I can identify and use words, phrases and sentence patterns related to the topic.	☐
I can write a letter telling one doctor-patient story using the terminologies and medical information in this unit.	☐
I understand how narrative medicine affects doctor-patient relationship.	☐

Unit 8
Artificial Intelligence and Medicine

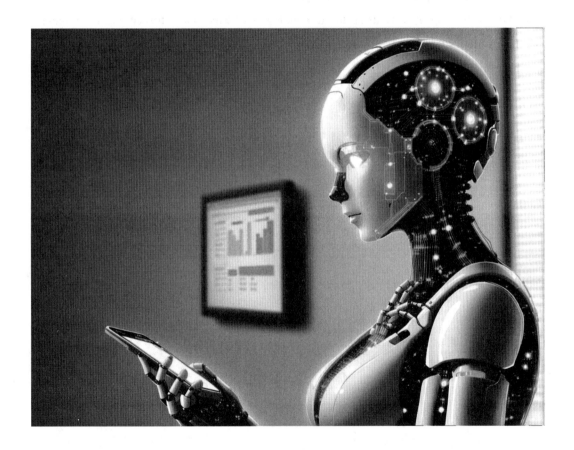

The term "artificial intelligence" means a machine-based system that can, for a given set of human-defined objectives, make predictions, recommendations or decisions influencing real or virtual environments. The development of AI has led to transformative advances now impacting our everyday lives. Properly designed AI has the potential to make our health care system more efficient and less expensive,

Lead in

211

ease the paperwork burden, fill the gaping holes in access to quality care in the world's poorest places, and, among many other things, serve as an unblinking watchdog on the lookout for the medical errors. Though the promise is great, the road ahead isn't necessarily smooth. Even AI's most ardent supporters acknowledge that the likely bumps and potholes, both seen and unseen, should be taken seriously.

This unit is mainly to achieve the following objectives:

1) Have some basic knowledge on artificial intelligence and medicine;

2) Identify words, phrases and sentence patterns related to the topic;

3) Make a thinking map by using the terminologies and medical information in this unit;

4) Learn the spirit of innovation from doctors and scientists who make contributions to the betterment of mankind.

Part I   View the Medical World

Watch a video about an intelligent robot and choose the right answer.①

1. Which of the following is a feature that Pepper does Not have?

    A. Behaving appropriately.

    B. Being available in multiple languages.

    C. Knowing the hospital environment well.

    F. Making accurate diagnoses.

2. What is the height of Pepper?

    A. 1. 2 meters.   B. 120 meters.

    C. 102 centimeters.   D. 20 centimeters.

3. What does Pepper need to function well?

    A. A leather jacket.   B. Internet access.

    C. A computer specialist.   D. Charging cable.

4. What is the maximum time the robot can work when the battery is fully charged?

    A. 20 hours.   B. 24 hours.

    C. More than one day.   D. More than one week.

5. Which of the following is true about Pepper's use in hospital?

    A. The mother was very anxious when Pepper was sent to the maternity ward.

    B. Pepper can walk at a mellow pace of 5 kilometers per hour.

    C. Pepper is able to cheer patients up.

    D. The baby got a shock the first time he saw Pepper.

---

① 视频详见网站:https://pan-yz. cldisk. com/external/m/file/1055138682145771520。

▣ Words and Phrases

humanoid /ˈhjuːmənɔɪd/ *adj.* 有人的特点的

manner /ˈmænə(r)/ *n.* 举止；态度

leather /ˈleðə(r)/ *n.* 皮；皮革；皮革制品

charge /tʃɑːdʒ/ *n.* 充电量

mellow /ˈmeləʊ/ *adj.* 稳健的

assign /əˈsaɪn/ *v.* 指定；指派

maternity ward /məˈtɜːnəti ˈwɔːd/ 产科病房；产房

reassure /ˌriːəˈʃʊə(r)/ *v.* 使……安心；打消……的疑虑

Part II Read to Explore Medical Knowledge

Text A

Pre-reading Questions:

1. As someone who will be working in the health care field, what do you expect AI to be able to do for you?

2. What do you think humans need to pay special attention to while developing AI?

Ten Best Ways Artificial Intelligence Could Enhance My Medical Practice

Text A

1. In the near future, artificial intelligence (AI) will completely revolutionize health care systems, but it will also have a positive influence on the "average doctor's" life. I'll outline ten ways AI could improve my work. Upon rewatching the film *Her*, I found myself intrigued by the sequence where Joaquin Phoenix's character receives his new AI operating system and begins to use it. I was obsessed with the idea of using an AI system in my life and how it would improve my practice as a doctor. It would be a big step toward improving if I could give patients the time it currently takes to cope with technology (entering data, searching for documents, etc.).

2. AI has the potential to enhance my abilities as a doctor in the following ten areas.

Minimizing the Duration of Waiting

3. It may be assumed that waiting is the exclusive "privilege" that only patients enjoy, while doctors have no free time during their overpacked days. Suboptimal health care processes lead to both patients experiencing prolonged waiting periods in front of doctors' offices and

medical professionals wasting significant amounts of time each day waiting for various factors such as patients or test results. An AI system that optimizes my schedule by guiding me to the most logical assignment would be a jackpot.

Arrange My E-mails in Order of Importance

4. We are currently seeing a significant and overwhelming tsunami of digital advancements. Our email inboxes are full of unopened messages, posing a daily struggle to avoid becoming overwhelmed by the deluge of new correspondence. I handle over 200 emails on a daily basis. There were three thousand unopened emails, but the AI system in *Her* quickly sorted them all. Think about how much easier and more effective it would be if digital communication were in line with our specific needs, allowing us to send and receive information with pinpoint accuracy and no effort.

Locate the Data I Require

5. I believe I have achieved proficiency in utilizing several Google search operators and diverse search engines for distinct purposes when seeking information online, however it still requires a considerable amount of effort. Imagine an AI operating system that could provide instant answers to my inquiries by searching for the information online. Both HealthTap and Your. Md aim to utilize AI to assist people in finding solutions for their most prevalent illnesses.

Keep Me Up-to-date

6. There is an excessive amount of information available. Without a suitable compass, we get disoriented and unable to navigate through the vast amount of information. It is crucial to locate the most precise, relevant, and current data.

7. Twenty-three million papers are available on PubMed. Even if I could read three or four studies related to my field of interest every week, I still wouldn't have time to study them all, especially considering the constant stream of new research that comes out. There will soon be an AI that can go through the mountain of data and present me with the papers that are most pertinent to my problem. A million pages can be processed in seconds by IBM Watson. Due to its impressive speed, Watson is now being tested at oncology centers to

assess its usefulness in cancer treatment decision-making.

Perform My Duties When I Don't

8. Using a desktop computer, laptop, or smartphone, I am able to complete all of my online chores, including checking email, reading papers, and conducting research. Obviously, I am unable to work when I am without any of these. If I were to lose my device, an AI system could handle these tasks.

9. Envision yourself engaged in a game of tennis or carrying out household chores when significant communication arrives. Utilizing AI, you can reply to your employer without the necessity of interacting with any devices, effectively managing the entire book publishing process on his behalf, without requiring any effort from him.

Assist Me in Making Difficult Decisions Sensible

10. On a daily basis, a doctor is faced with a series of challenging decisions. Making well-informed selections is our best option. Basically, the only thing I can do is asking people whose opinions I respect. Regretfully, you would look up specific answers on the internet in vain.

11. However, systems driven by AI may prove useful down the road. As an illustration, IBM Watson launched its unique program for oncologists, about which I spoke with a professor. This tool enables professionals to access evidence-based treatment alternatives. Advanced data analysis capabilities in Watson for Oncology allow it to make sense of clinical notes and reports containing both structured and unstructured data, which could be essential when choosing a treatment course. Thus, AI does not make the diagnosis decision but rather presents you with the most reasonable alternatives.

Make It Easier for Patients to Contact Me in an Emergency

12. On a regular basis, a doctor receives a large volume of calls, inquiries from patients, emails, and even messages from social media platforms. Amidst all this data, not every critical issue would be able to reach you. What if, instead of sifting through all the chaos, an AI operation system could pick out the most important ones and bring them to your notice when they're really needed?

Aid Me in Becoming Better Over Time

13. People, no matter how hard they try, inevitably make the same mistakes. Imagine I could do a better job if I talked to an AI about every challenging decision or assignment. Take a quick look at this:

14. Zorgprisma Publiek, a local business in the Netherlands, handles the data via IBM Watson in the cloud. They can assist medical facilities improve patient care and reduce avoidable hospitalizations by identifying when doctors, clinics, or hospitals make the same mistakes when treating the same conditions.

Allow Me to Collaborate More

15. Occasionally, I ponder the number of researchers, doctors, nurses, or patients who contemplate the same health care challenges as I do. During those moments, I see having an AI companion that assists me in identifying the most promising collaborators and extending invitations to collaborate towards a better future. Establishing clinical and scientific collaborations is essential for identifying optimal solutions to arising problems. However, more often than not, it is challenging to identify the most appropriate partners.

Perform Administrative Tasks

16. A significant portion of a doctor's usual day is devoted to administrative tasks. An AI has the potential to acquire the necessary skills and perform the task more effectively than me over time. The health care sector is particularly susceptible to significant influence from AI in this particular domain. AI should be utilized to perform mundane and monotonous jobs that do not require any level of creativity. IBM introduced a new technology called Medical Sieve. The project aims to construct a sophisticated "cognitive assistant" that possesses advanced analytical and reasoning abilities, as well as extensive therapeutic knowledge. This endeavor is characterized by its ambitious nature and long-term scope.

17. There is widespread concern that AI will replace the employment of medical professionals in the future. I am quite skeptical. AI will augment medical professionals rather than replace them. By eliminating the day-to-day treadmill of administrative and repetitive duties, the medical community would be able to fully dedicate their attention to their primary objective: healing.

✍ New Words and Expressions

artificial intelligence the simulation of human intelligence in machines that are designed to think and act like humans 人工智能

AI operating system a specialized operating system designed to support and enhance the capabilities of artificial intelligence applications and services 人工智能操作系统

exclusive /ɪkˈskluːsɪv/ *adj.* only to be used by one particular person or group; only given to one particular person or group (个人或集体)专用的; 专有的; 独有的; 独占的

privilege /ˈprɪvəlɪdʒ/ *n.* a special right or advantage that a particular person or group of people has 特殊利益; 优惠待遇

overpacked /ˈəʊvəˈpækt/ *adj.* loaded past capacity 超载的; 负荷过重的

suboptimal /ˈsʌbˈɒptɪməl/ *adj.* not at the best possible level 未达最佳标准的; 不最理想的; 不最适宜的; 不最满意的

medical professional an individual who has received specialized education and training in the field of medicine and provides health care services to patients 医疗专业人员

jackpot /ˈdʒækpɒt/ *n.* a large amount of money that is the most valuable prize in a game of chance (在碰运气游戏中的)头奖; 最高奖

tsunami /tsuːˈnɑːmi/ *n.* an extremely large wave in the sea caused, for example, by an earthquake 海啸; 海震

in line with used to indicate that something is consistent with, or in agreement with, another thing 符合; 与……一致

aim /eɪm/ *v.* to try or plan to achieve sth. 力求达到; 力争做到

up-to-date /ˌʌp tə ˈdeɪt/ *adj.* reflecting the latest information or changes 包含最新信息的; 新式的

compass /ˈkʌmpəs/ *n.* a range or an extent, especially of what can be achieved in a particular situation 范围; 范畴; 界限

process /ˈprəʊses/ *v.* to perform a series of operations on data in a computer 数据处理

device /dɪˈvaɪs/ *n.* an object or a piece of equipment that has been designed to do a particular job 装置; 仪器; 器具; 设备

a series of used to indicate a sequence or succession of related events, objects, actions, or occurrences 一系列

in vain without success or to no avail 徒劳无益地；无用地

launch /lɔːntʃ/ v. to start an activity, especially an organized one 开始从事；发起；发动（尤指有组织的活动）

unstructured /ʌnˈstrʌktʃəd/ adj. without structure or organization 结构凌乱的；无条理的；紊乱的；无序的

condition /kənˈdɪʃn/ n. an illness or a medical problem that you have for a long time because it is not possible to cure it（因不可能治愈而长期患有的）疾病

collaborate /kəˈlæbəreɪt/ v. to work together with sb. in order to produce or achieve sth. 合作；协作

arising /əˈraɪzɪŋ/ adj. happening, starting to exist 发生的；出现的

more often than not used to indicate that something happens frequently or with a high probability 往往；多半

monotonous /məˈnɒtənəs/ adj. never changing and therefore boring 单调乏味的

reasoning /ˈriːzənɪŋ/ n. the process of thinking about things in a logical way; opinions and ideas that are based on logical thinking 推想；推理；理性的观点；论证

augment /ɔːɡˈment/ v. to increase the amount, value, size, etc. of sth. 增加；提高；扩大

treadmill /ˈtredmɪl/ n. work or a way of life that is boring or tiring because it involves always doing the same things 枯燥无味的工作(或生活方式)

medical community a collective group of health care professionals and institutions involved in the field of medicine 医学界

▤ Notes

1. PubMed：It is a free resource supporting the search and retrieval of biomedical and life sciences literature with the aim of improving health—both globally and personally. The PubMed database contains more than 36 million citations and abstracts of biomedical literature.

　　PubMed 是一个支持搜索和检索生物医学和生命科学文献的免费资源库，旨在改善全

球和个人的健康状况。PubMed 数据库包含 3600 多万条生物医学文献的引文和摘要。

2. IBM Watson：The supercomputer "Watson" was jointly built by IBM and the University of Texas over a period of four years. The computer stores huge amounts of data and has a logical reasoning program that can reason out what it thinks is the most correct answer. Watson was taken in honor of IBM founder Thomas J. Watson. IBM developed Watson to fulfill a daunting challenge：to build a computing system that rivals a human's ability to answer questions.

超级电脑"沃森"由国际商业机器公司（IBM）和美国得克萨斯大学历时四年联合打造，电脑存储了海量的数据，而且拥有一套逻辑推理程序，可以推理出它认为最正确的答案。沃森（Watson）是为了纪念 IBM 创始人托马期·J. 沃森（Thomas J. Watson）而得名。IBM 开发沃森旨在完成一项艰巨挑战：建造一个能与人类回答问题能力匹敌的计算系统。

After Reading Activities

Reading Comprehension

I. Answer the following questions.

1. How can AI system help both patients and doctors reduce waiting time？

2. Why is IBM Watson applied in hospitals for treating cancer？

3. How can IBM Watson help clinicians choose a treatment course？

4. What is the area where AI could impact health care the most？

5. According to the text, what will the relationship between artificial intelligence and doctors be like in the future？

II. Work in groups to complete the following chart according to the structure of the text.

Introduction：(para. 1)

Artificial intelligence（AI）will completely revolutionize _____ in the near future, but it will also impact the life of _____ positively.

Body part：(paras. 2-16)

Through the following ten ways, AI could make me a better doctor.

Minimizing the Duration of Waiting

Suboptimal health care processes not only result in ＿＿＿＿＿＿ experiencing prolonged waiting periods in front of doctors' offices but also ＿＿＿＿＿＿＿＿＿ losing a lot of time everyday waiting for something (a patient, a lab result, etc.). An AI system can make doctors' schedule as efficient as possible.

Arrange My E-mails in Order of Importance

Do digital communication completely ＿＿＿＿＿＿ our needs. Send and receive information with ＿＿＿＿＿＿＿＿＿ and no effort.

Locate the Data I Require

＿＿＿＿＿＿＿＿＿ could answer my questions immediately by searching for the information online.

Keep Me Up-to-date

I need an AI that can go through the mountain of data and present me with the papers that are most ＿＿＿＿＿＿＿＿ to my problem.

Perform My Duties When I Don't

If I were to lose my ＿＿＿＿＿＿, an AI system could handle my tasks.

Assist Me in Making Difficult Decisions Sensible

AI is not making the ＿＿＿＿＿＿ decision but rather presents you with the most reasonable alternatives.

Make It Easier for Patients to Contact Me in an Emergency

AI operation system could pick out the key information from the mess and bring it to the doctor's ＿＿＿＿＿＿ when it is really needed.

Aid Me in Becoming Better Over Time

By discussing every ＿＿＿＿＿＿ decision or assignment with AI, doctors can improve the quality of their work.

Allow Me to Collaborate More

AI could assist health care professionals in identifying the most promising collaborators and ＿＿＿＿＿＿＿＿＿ towards a better future.

Perform Administrative Tasks

An AI could learn how to do ＿＿＿＿＿＿＿＿＿ stuff properly and do it better than the medical professionals over time.

Conclusion：(para. 17)

　　AI will ＿＿＿＿＿＿ doctors rather than replace them. Without the repetitive administrative tasks, the medical community could focus on its most important task with full attention：＿＿＿＿＿＿.

Words and Phrases

✅ I. Translate the following medical terms into Chinese or English.

1. medical professional　　＿＿＿＿＿＿＿＿＿＿＿＿＿＿

2. cognitive assistant　　＿＿＿＿＿＿＿＿＿＿＿＿＿＿

3. medical community　　＿＿＿＿＿＿＿＿＿＿＿＿＿＿

4. treat the condition　　＿＿＿＿＿＿＿＿＿＿＿＿＿＿

5. 人工智能操作系统　　＿＿＿＿＿＿＿＿＿＿＿＿＿＿

6. 肿瘤中心　　＿＿＿＿＿＿＿＿＿＿＿＿＿＿

7. 临床报告　　＿＿＿＿＿＿＿＿＿＿＿＿＿＿

8. 治疗方案　　＿＿＿＿＿＿＿＿＿＿＿＿＿＿

✅ II. Fill in the blanks with the words or phrases given below. Change the form if necessary.

privilege	monotonous	clinical	condition	suboptimal

1. ＿＿＿＿＿＿ health is the state between health and disease. There is an increasing number of individuals worldwide who report a general malaise even in the absence of a diagnosable disorder.

2. She enjoys her ＿＿＿＿＿＿ practice but is looking forward to working in a laboratory as doing research is what she does best.

3. Many people paint rosy picture of the explorers' lives, but they lived on a ＿＿＿＿＿＿ diet of beans and rice.

4. The company's executives were granted the ＿＿＿＿＿＿ of flying business class on all company-sponsored travel.

5. He was admitted to the hospital this morning with a heart attack and was reported to be in

critical _____ .

Sentence Translation

Translate the following sentences into Chinese or English.

1. Suboptimal health care processes lead to both patients experiencing prolonged waiting periods in front of doctors' offices and medical professionals wasting significant amounts of time each day waiting for various factors such as patients or test results.

   _____

   _____

2. They can assist medical facilities improve patient care and reduce avoidable hospitalizations by identifying when doctors, clinics, or hospitals make the same mistakes when treating the same conditions.

   _____

   _____

3. The project aims to construct a sophisticated "cognitive assistant" that possesses advanced analytical and reasoning abilities, as well as an extensive therapeutic knowledge.

   _____

   _____

4. 想一想，如果数字通信能够满足我们的特定需求，让我们能够准确无误地发送和接收信息，该是有多么方便和高效啊。

   _____

   _____

5. 先进的数据分析功能使其能够理解包含结构化和非结构化数据的临床笔记和报告，这对选择治疗方案至关重要。

   _____

   _____

Text B

Pre-reading Questions:

1. Can you list the things that AI can do in medicine?

2. Do you know any drawbacks of AI being used in medicine?

How Health Care Is Being Shaped by AI

Text B

1. The ability to analyze a pathology report for cancer discoveries in only a quarter of a second may not seem like a significant inprovement. But when compared to the typical time it takes a person to read such a report, which is 90 seconds to 3 minutes, it becomes apparent. That speedy reading was courtesy of artificial intelligence (AI) technology from Azra AI. *Journal of Clinical Oncology* findings show that the tech saved 11,141 hours of manual labor over three months, which is equivalent to 1,392 eight-hour days. Treatment time was also reduced by 7 days for patients.

2. AI is transforming medicine and health care, and experts anticipate that its effect will be much more monumental in the upcoming years, despite the hurdles it may face.

The Internal Brain

3. AI may first seem complex, particularly if you lack technical expertise. However, if you have ever interacted with Siri on your iPhone or used a robot vacuum, you are already acquainted with AI. But what is it precisely? The textbook definition is an intelligent agent capable of accomplishing a goal determined by humans according to Lurong Pan, PhD, founder and CEO of Ainnocence, a global biotech startup. Ainnocence is using an AI-driven drug-design platform to expedite the creation of novel drugs. "AI, at its most basic level, is an expert system capable of substituting a specific degree of work performed by experts," Pan explains. At the advanced level, AI has the capability to accomplish technological advancements that surpass the abilities of specialists or scientists.

4. In order to do this, AI technology goes through a learning process that is comparable to the

human learning experience. "Children acquire knowledge through the process of providing information and repeating it, and computers acquire knowledge in a similar way," said Connor Landgraf, the CEO and co-founder of Eko. The company was responsible for developing the first stethoscope driven by AI.

5. For example, Eko feeds its AI systems hundreds of heart sounds, enabling them to differentiate between normal heart sounds and those that may suggest issues such as a heart murmur. After a few uses, the stethoscope's algorithm learns to differentiate between heart sounds autonomously, enabling the stethoscope to rapidly screen for heart illness within a just 15-second timeframe. Additionally, Landgraf asserts that it is not only quicker but also more precise than people. Thousands of doctors are already using the AI stethoscope; it even helps in nations with fewer resources, where health care workers may examine patients and send the heart sounds to a distant specialist, enabling them to assess as many as 2,000 individuals daily.

6. Pan is unsurprised by AI's cognitive powers and remarks that its imagination is enormous. "The imaginary space of it surpasses that of humans," she explains, referring to the ongoing efforts of medicinal chemists in developing new small-molecule drugs, which are compounds with low molecular weight. These medications are commonly available in everyone's medical cabinet and include aspirin and the antihistamine diphenhydramine (Benadryl).

7. In order to locate a single molecule suitable for clinical trials, scientists doing the testing by themselves must undertake around 6,000 experiments. But with AI, that number drops to about 150. According to Pan, the drugs eventually reach the patient faster and at a cheaper price since fewer molecules are evaluated before they reach clinical stage, which means less time and money spent.

Beneficial Outcomes

8. For the last 5 years, or even longer in the case of medication development, the health care business has been using AI. According to Chris Cashwell, CEO and creator of Azra AI, whose technology is used in 200 hospitals throughout the U.S., "It's possible that the average consumer may not be aware that AI is being used behind the scenes in a whole host of areas."

9. While AI has many potential uses, one study published in the *Journal of Family Medicine and Primary Care* found that it is most commonly employed in the following areas of health care: developing drugs, diagnosing diseases, analyzing health plans, monitoring health, providing digital consultations, performing surgeries, managing medical data and personalized medicine.

10. Despite the fact that 15.1% of all general procedures were done robotically as of 2018, a 2020 analysis of almost 170,000 patients published in *JAMA Network Open* suggests that hospitals will not one day be staffed entirely by robots. AI still requires human oversight. However, AI has the potential to enhance human productivity and work performance, which would benefit the cost-conscious health care system, doctors, and patients above all. An essential benefit of AI, according to Cashwell, is that it frees up doctors to spend more time with patients and less time processing data.

11. A research published in *JAMA Network Open* examined the potential of an AI system to enhance clinicians' proficiency in extracting patient information from electronic health records (EHR). The AI solution not only improved accuracy, but also reduced physicians' review time of patients' records by 20%. This time savings may be allocated towards patient visits, since doctors typically examine health data prior to each consultation.

12. Although it may not seem significant, experts assert that the accumulated savings might be substantial over time for each patient. According to Ethan A. Chi, co-author of the *JAMA* paper and a recent graduate of Stanford University, AI-augmented EHR systems have the potential to save time, minimize errors, and even synthesize together disparate information to assist clinicians. For instance, an AI-backed EHR system may identify a potential adverse medication interaction or indicate an uncommon disease that doctors overlooked.

Potential Outcomes for the Future

13. Health care and medication development have already been profoundly affected by AI, but scientists predict that this influence will only grow in the future. Pan holds the opinion that AI will play a pivotal role in finding treatments for the approximately 10,000 illnesses that now lack them, with 8,000 of them being uncommon genetic disorders. "Considerably, we can expedite the diagnostics of these diseases and discover treatments for them with the

assistance of AI," she remarks. She goes on to say that the goal is to make therapy more accessible by reducing the time and expense of medication development for each of these illnesses by 50% to 80%.

14. Cashwell from Azra AI supports it. "As we gather more data on individuals and develop more treatments that specifically target personal traits, health care will become increasingly personalized," he asserts. Regarding cancer therapy, it is seen that Azra is making progress in enhancing the identification of incidental discoveries. These are outcomes discovered during a medical test that a doctor requests, but are unrelated to the initial purpose of the test, for example, a nodule on the lung is detected during an abdominal CT scan.

15. AI can enhance the detection, tracking, and monitoring of these cases. "The objective is to ensure that individuals receive appropriate medical treatment, thereby preventing them from returning a year later with stage 3 cancer instead of undergoing a minor procedure to remove a nodule," said Cashwell. AI has the ability to provide improved criteria for determining whether an incidental discovery does not need further investigation, which might possibly decrease unnecessary medical interventions.

16. According to Eko's Landgraf, there is room for innovation in home AI devices. "Instead of going to a doctor's office for a heart or lung exam, people with these conditions may one day be able to do it remotely, just like you can take your blood pressure readings at home with a blood pressure cuff," he adds.

17. However, it is important to note that AI is not without its downsides. One important aspect is that it mostly relies on data. The issue lies in the limited application area of the data due to its poor quality, as stated by Pan. To put it another, if the input data is of poor quality, the output data will also be of poor quality.

18. Some individuals are worried by technology since it is not readily explained or trusted. Scientists have a hard time trusting AI as "most AI is a black box of knowledge that cannot be explained by conventional chemistry or biology rules," as Pan puts it. That might explain why some medical organizations and doctors are hesitant to adopt AI. The fear of losing their employment is another possible explanation.

19. It is also only the beginning, even if its potential is encouraging. AI alone may be able to predict how health care will develop in the future.

New Words and Expressions

courtesy /ˈkɜːtəsi/ *n.* polite behaviour that shows respect for other people 礼貌；谦恭；彬彬有礼

manual /ˈmænjuəl/ *adj.* involving using the hands or physical strength 用手的；手工的；体力的

monumental /ˌmɒnjuˈmentl/ *adj.* very important and having a great influence, especially as the result of years of work 重要的；意义深远的；不朽的

upcoming /ˈʌpkʌmɪŋ/ *adj.* going to happen soon 即将发生（或来临）的

robot vacuum an autonomous domestic appliance designed to clean floors without human intervention 扫地机器人

startup /ˈstɑːtʌp/ *n.* a small business that has recently been started by someone 新兴公司；新开张的企业

expedite /ˈekspədaɪt/ *v.* to make a process happen more quickly 加快；加速

stethoscope /ˈsteθəskəʊp/ *n.* an instrument that a doctor uses to listen to sb.'s heart and breathing 听诊器

heart murmur an unusual sound heard during a heartbeat 心脏杂音

algorithm /ˈælgərɪðəm/ *n.* a set of rules that must be followed when solving a particular problem 算法；计算程序

screen /skriːn/ *v.* to examine people in order to find out if they have a particular disease or illness 筛查；检查

specialist /ˈspeʃəlɪst/ *n.* a doctor who has specialized in a particular area of medicine 专科医生

assess /əˈses/ *v.* to make a judgement about the nature or quality of sb./sth. 评估，评定（性质、质量）

medicinal /məˈdɪsɪnl/ *adj.* helpful in the process of healing illness or infection 有疗效的；药用的；药的

small-molecule drug a type of pharmaceutical agent that is composed of relatively small molecules, typically with molecular weights below 1000 Daltons 小分子药物

molecular /məˈlekjələ(r)/ *adj.* relating to or produced by or consisting of molecules 分子的，由分子组成的

aspirin /ˈæsprɪn/ *n.* a drug used to reduce pain, fever and inflammation 阿司匹林(镇痛解热消炎药)

a whole host of a large number or a great variety of something 大量

cost-conscious /ˈkɒstkˈɒnʃəs/ *adj.* aware of the cost 注重节约成本的

extract /ɪkˈstrækt/ *v.* to choose information, etc. from a book, a computer, etc. to be used for a particular purpose 选取；摘录；选录

savings /ˈseɪvɪŋz/ *n.* (plural noun) an economy of or reduction in money, time, or another resource 节省物；节省；节约

synthesize /ˈsɪnθəsaɪz/ *v.* to combine separate ideas, beliefs, styles, etc. 综合

disparate /ˈdɪspərət/ *adj.* essentially different in kind; not allowing comparison 完全不同的

AI-backed *adj.* supported by artificial intelligence 人工智能技术支持的

target /ˈtɑːɡɪt/ *v.* to try to have an effect on a particular group of people 面向；把……对准(某群体)

incidental /ˌɪnsɪˈdentl/ *adj.* happening in connection with sth. else, but not as important as it, or not intended 附带发生的；次要的；非有意的

nodule /ˈnɒdjuːl/ *n.* a small round lump or swelling 节结；小瘤

blood pressure cuff a medical device used to measure the pressure of blood in the arteries [医]血压表套袖

📇 Notes

1. Azra AI：It is a high-tech company that uses artificial intelligence to help health care providers find at-risk patients that need cancer care.

　　Azra AI 是一家高科技公司，利用人工智能帮助医疗保健机构找到需要癌症治疗的高危患者。

2. *Journal of Clinical Oncology*：《临床肿瘤学杂志》

3. antihistamine diphenhydramine (Benadryl)：Antihistamine diphenhydramine (trade name：Benadryl) used to treat allergic reactions involving the nasal passages (hay fever) and also to treat motion sickness.

抗组胺药苯海拉明(商品名：Benadryl)，用于治疗鼻腔过敏反应(花粉热)和晕动病。

4. *Journal of Family Medicine and Primary Care*：《家庭医学与初级保健杂志》

5. *JAMA Network Open*：*JAMA Network Open* is an international, peer-reviewed, open access, general medical journal that publishes research on clinical care, innovation in health care, health policy, and global health across all health disciplines and countries for clinicians, investigators, and policy makers.

《美国医学会杂志(网络公开版)》是一本国际性、同行评审、开放获取的普通医学杂志，为临床医生、研究人员和政策制定者发布所有卫生学科和国家的以临床护理、医疗保健创新、卫生政策和全球健康为主题的研究文章。

▤ After Reading Activities

Reading Comprehension

Decide whether the following statements are true (T) or false (F) according to the text.

_____ 1. AI can save doctors' time to read medical reports and patients' time to treatment.

_____ 2. The AI stethoscope is even used in some developing countries to diagnose heart diseases efficiently.

_____ 3. One of the most important changes that artificial intelligence brings to doctors is that they need to spend more time processing data.

_____ 4. Artificial intelligence can solve the problem of over treatment thoroughly.

_____ 5. The more data being fed to the AI products, the more advanced they can be.

Words and Phrases

Match each English phrase in Column A with its Chinese version in Column B.

Column A	Column B
1. biotech startup	A. 心脏杂音
2. blood pressure cuff	B. 病理报告
3. electronic health record	C. 药物化学研究员
4. pathology report	D. 人工智能听诊器
5. AI-powered stethoscope	E. 电子病历
6. heart murmur	F. 血压表套袖
7. medicinal chemist	G. 临床期
8. clinical stage	H. 生物技术初创企业

Translation

　　今天进入人工智能发展阶段，大家经常会问，科技手段这么发达，可以解决这么多问题，人工智能是否会替代医生？人工智能可以提高医疗服务水平，但是不能替代医生。根据我们对医疗服务的定义，医疗服务不仅仅等于医疗技术服务，医疗服务是医疗技术加上医学人文。因为医学不仅仅是科学，更是社会学，所以医学人文的情怀是永恒的。我们让这些高科技产品，变得更有人文温度，就要把医学人文融入科技发展，尤其是融入人工智能发展。

_____

_____

_____

Critical Thinking

　　Currently, AI can diagnose patients and even perform surgeries remotely. But will this lead to a psychological gap between doctors and patients? Please work in groups to have a discussion focusing on how to bridge psychological gap between doctors and patients while AI is involved in medical treatment.

Part III　Apply Medical English

✅ A. Situational Dialogues in Different Clinical Departments

Emergency（急诊科）

Fracture（骨折）

Doctor：What's wrong with you?

Patient：My chest hurts a lot.

Doctor：When and how did it happen?

Patient：My car collided with another car about an hour ago. My chest hit the steering wheel hard. Then I felt a sharp pain in my chest. There must be something wrong with my ribs or lungs!

Doctor：OK, I will examine you. Please point out the place you feel most painful.

Patient：Here.

Doctor：Breathe deeply. Has the pain got worse?

Patient：Yes.

Doctor：Do you find it difficult to breathe?

Patient：No.

Doctor：OK. I'd like you to have an X-ray, and come back to me after you have had it.

Patient：Here is the X-ray and the result report, doctor.

Doctor：Well, there is a complicated fracture in your ribs, but your lung and heart seem to be normal. Don't worry. I will locate an orthopedist to fix your injured ribs.

Patient：Will it hurt much doctor?

Doctor：We will try to be very gentle with you, and we'll also give you a sedative before the procedure.

Patient：Thank you, doctor. This has been a very difficult day for me. I do appreciate your kindness and concern. I will try to be a good patient.

Doctor：Keep up the spirit. It will be all over before you know it. We will take good care of you.

Words and Phrases

steering wheel /ˈstɪərɪŋ wiːl/ 方向盘

rib /rɪb/ n. 肋骨

fracture /ˈfræktʃə(r)/ n. 骨折

orthopedist /ˌɔːθəuˈpiːdist/ n. 骨科医生

sedative /ˈsedətɪv/ n. 镇定药

keep up the spirit /kiːp ʌp ðə ˈspɪrɪt/ 振作起来

Notes

Here are top 10 most common ER diseases and what these symptoms could indicate.

Headaches

The number one and the most common ER visit is due to headaches. They are the most common ailments amongst people and it stands to reason that headaches are the most common reason for a person to visit the ER.

Foreign Objects in the Body

Emergency room centers all over the world report that one of the most common ER visits is due to foreign objects inside the body. There aren't any stats regarding the number of doctors that have to deal with foreign objects but a recent analysis has shown that there are roughly 1,500 deaths per year due to foreign object problems.

Skin Infections

Skin infections can cause abnormal reactions in the body and in the majority of cases they require urgent emergency care. A skin infection can also bring on other symptoms and can spread rapidly over the body in severe cases. Symptoms may include：

- Nerve damage
- Muscle weakness
- Lesions on the body
- Rashes and blisters

Back Pain

Back pains or muscle strains in the back can be due to an accident or physical injuries while playing sports or by lifting heavy things.

Contusions and Cuts

Cuts and contusions are one of the most common reasons why people visit the ER. They can occur through any activity and often require urgent emergency attention. The majority of cuts and contusions are due to accidents with a glass or a knife and in case of severe bleeding.

Upper Respiratory Infections

Infections and viruses are another common cause of people visiting the ER. The flu and common cold are fairly widespread diseases and unlike other illnesses, may require emergency treatment in severe cases if related to fever.

Broken Bones and Sprains

Broken bones and sprains are a common occurrence that can happen to any individual regardless of their age or condition. They can be caused due to accidents or twisting an area of the body while playing sports or other physical activities. Not all sprains require ER treatment although broken bones need to be looked at immediately, particularly if they pose a risk to other organs. Some key ways to determine if the injury needs medical attention are:

- Discoloration
- Swelling
- Visible bone

Toothaches

Most people will not relate tooth-related issues with the ER, but an increasing number of people are pursuing emergency treatments when dentist offices are closed. The majority of patients report abscesses, and gum tissues problems.

Abdominal Pains

Around 2000 people visit the ER every single day due to abdominal pains. Most likely, bacterial and viral infections are the cause of abdominal pains. The culprit of abdominal pains can be a factor to several different diagnoses.

- Food Poisoning/Allergies
- Kidney Stones
- Stomach Virus

- Appendicitis
- Ulcers
- Irritable Bowel Syndrome

Chest Pains

Chest pains are one of the most common reasons why people visit the ER. Cardiac arrest situations are common in the ER and although chest pain visits are declining in recent years, still nearly half a million people die each year due to heart complications.

以下是前十大常见急诊疾病及其症状可能暗示的问题。

头痛：

头痛是人们去急诊室的最常见原因之一。它们是最常见的疾病之一，因此，头痛成为人们访问急诊室的主要原因。

体内异物：

世界各地的急诊室报告显示，体内异物是常见的急诊原因之一。目前没有关于医生处理体内异物数量的统计数据，但最近的分析表明，每年大约有 1500 人因异物问题死亡。

皮肤感染：

皮肤感染会导致身体出现异常反应，多数情况下需要紧急治疗。皮肤感染还可能引发其他症状，严重时可迅速蔓延。症状可能包括：神经损伤、肌肉无力、皮肤病变、皮疹和水疱。

背痛：

背痛或背部肌肉拉伤可能是由于突发事故或体育活动中受伤引起的。

挫伤和割伤：

挫伤和割伤是人们去急诊的常见原因之一。它们可能由任何活动引起，通常需要紧急处理。大多数挫割伤是由玻璃或刀具引起的事故，如果出现出血严重的情况，就需要去急诊室就诊。

上呼吸道感染：

感染和病毒是人们去急诊的另一常见原因。流感和普通感冒是较为普遍的疾病，在严重情况下，尤其是伴发高烧，可能需要急诊治疗。

骨折和扭伤：

骨折和扭伤是常见的急诊原因，任何年龄或身体状况的人都可能发生。它们通常是由事故、运动或其他体力活动中的扭伤引起的。并非所有扭伤都需要急诊治疗，但骨折特别是如果对其他器官构成威胁时需要立即处理。判断伤情是否需要医疗护理的关键是：变色、肿胀、骨骼外露。

牙痛：

大多数人不会将牙齿问题与急诊联系起来，但越来越多的人在牙科诊所关闭时寻求急诊治疗。大多数患者要求处理牙龈脓肿和牙龈组织问题。

腹痛：

每天约有 2000 人因腹痛前往急诊室就诊。腹痛最可能的原因是细菌和病毒感染。腹痛的罪魁祸首可能与几种不同的诊断有关，包括：食物中毒/过敏、肾结石、胃病毒、阑尾炎、溃疡、肠易激综合征。

胸痛：

胸痛是人们去急诊的常见原因之一。心脏骤停在急诊室中很常见，尽管近年来胸痛就诊数量有所下降，但每年仍有近 50 万人因心脏并发症死亡。

Practical Activity

Work with your partner to create and perform a doctor-patient dialogue related to common diseases in emergency department.

B. Practical Unit Project

Working in groups to have a discussion and draw a mind map on whether the intelligent robots will replace human doctors in the future.

Guidance for Production

Tips for having a discussion：

Step 1：Decide on your stand.

- Do you like intelligent robot? Why?
- What are the differences between intelligent robot and human doctor?
- Does intelligent robot bring more positives or negatives?

Step 2：Collect information or evidence to support your point of view.

Supporting details are essential to convincing argument.

The supporting information may come from：

personal experiences, memories, observations, hypothetical examples, reasoned arguments, facts, statistics, testimony from authorities, research, etc..

Step 3: Discuss your ideas with your group members.

Try not to be offensive.

Expressions for discussion:

I'm afraid that... / I think it would be better that... / Is it possible that...

Tips for making a mind map:

Step 1: Begin with the main concept.

Your main concept is your point of view on the topic.

Step 2: Add branches to the main concept.

The branches are your basic subtopics.

Step 3: Explore topics by adding more branches.

These branches are your supporting details of the subtopics.

Step 4: Add images and colors.

Maintain organization within your mind map by using standard colors for the different levels of thoughts. Furthermore, using images will help you both visualize, and memorize the various parts of your mind map.

Part IV   Self-Assessment

Use the following self-assessment checklist to check what you have learned in this unit.

I have some basic knowledge on artificial intelligence and medicine.	☐
I can identify and use words, phrases and sentence patterns related to the topic.	☐
I can make a thinking map by using the terminologies and medical information in this unit with my group members.	☐
I understand the spirit of innovation from doctors and scientists who make contributions to the betterment of mankind.	☐

Unit 1　Keys to Exercises and Audio Scripts

Part I　View the Medical World

1. B　2. A　3. C　4. D　5. D

Script

Ebola is one of the deadliest viruses we know of. If left untreated, it kills about half of those it infects. It can spread through pretty much every fluid your body makes, including blood and sweat. Even the dead can transmit the disease, often doing so at their own funerals. On December 26th, 2013, a two-year-old boy in southern Guinea got sick. Just two days later, he died. It took local doctors working with the international community four months to discover that Ebola was to blame, largely because it had never before been detected outside of Central Africa. In those four months, Ebola gained a head start that would prove devastating. The outbreak lasted two years and mushroomed into the largest Ebola epidemic in recorded history. More than 28,000 people contracted the disease and over 11,000 died. In 2013, Guinea had no formal emergency response system, few trained contact tracers, and no rapid tests, border screenings, or licensed vaccine for Ebola. After that epidemic, Guinea, with the support of the U.S. and other international partners, completely overhauled their epidemic response system. And in January 2021, that system faced its first real test. It started when a nurse in southern Guinea developed a headache, vomiting, and fever. A few days later, she died. As dictated by traditional burial practices, her family prepared her body for the funeral. Within a week, the nurse's husband and other family members started experiencing symptoms. Health officials suspected Ebola much quicker than in 2013 and ordered tests. They came back positive, and Guinea activated its epidemic alert system the next day. Then, lots of things happened very quickly. Guinea's National Agency for Health Security activated 38 district-level emergency operations centers, as well as a national one. Teams of epidemiologists and contact tracers began the painstaking job of figuring out exactly who was exposed and when, generating a list of 23 initial contacts that quickly grew to over 1,100. Advanced rapid testing capacity spun up in the city where the outbreak started. At Guinea's borders with Liberia and Cote d'Ivoire, public health workers screened more than 2 million travelers. A large-scale vaccination campaign was started. And, finally, more than 900 community mobilizers alerted people of the outbreak and suggested alternative burial practices that were acceptable to the community and reduced the risk of spreading Ebola. Thanks to all these measures, the 2021 outbreak ended just four months after it began. Only 23 people contracted Ebola; only 12 died. That's less than 1% of the deaths in the prior outbreak. The 2021 outbreak cost $100 million to control—which sounds like a lot but pales in comparison to the global economic cost of the previous outbreak: $53 billion.

Part II   Read to Explore Medical Knowledge

Text A

After Reading Activities

Reading Comprehension

Ⅰ. Answer the following questions.

1. The morbidity and mortality linked to SARS-CoV-2 have significantly decreased due to the combination of immunity obtained from vaccination and infections, together with the widespread availability of rapid diagnostics and effective therapies. Since most people have long handled influenza and other respiratory viruses without feeling compelled to mask, the majority of SARS-CoV-2 infections are currently no more severe than those infections.

2. To begin with, hospitals aggregate some of the most vulnerable people in society when they are at heightened vulnerability. These people still face an elevated risk of severe illness and death. Furthermore, it is important to note that nosocomial infections caused by respiratory viruses, excluding SARS-CoV-2, are frequently occurring but often not fully acknowledged. Additionally, the potential adverse health consequences linked to these viruses in susceptible patients are often underestimated.

3. Medical professionals can prevent around 60% of nosocomial respiratory viral infections by using masks, according to studies conducted before and during the pandemic.

4. The proposed strategy involves connecting masking requirements judiciously to community viral transmission levels, workers' current activities, and individual patients' risk of severe sickness.

5. Patients at particularly high risk for poor outcomes from respiratory viral infections should be advised to wear masks themselves in higher-risk situations year-round.

II. Work in groups to complete the following chart according to the structure of the text.

The current situation：(paras. 1-2)

the implementation of universal masking, source control, exposure protection, Ceasing the use of masks

The necessities of masking application in health care facilities：(paras. 3-5)

vulnerable, Nosocomial infections, known and unknown

Solutions to apply masking requirements judiciously：(paras. 6-9)

masking fatigue, surveillance metrics, predetermined months, Not every situation, masking all year round, poor outcomes

Conclusion：(para. 10)

reimagine their current approach to masking

Words and Phrases

I. Translate the following medical terms into Chinese or English.

1. 呼吸道病毒感染

5. asymptomatic infection

2. 医疗机构

6. surveillance metrics

3. 免疫功能受损的状况

7. community transmission

4. 阻塞性肺病

8. public health

II. Fill in the blanks with the words or phrases given below. Change the form if necessary.

1. triggers

4. adverse

2. aggregated

5. exposure

3. circulated

Sentence Translation

1. 由于疫苗接种和感染产生了免疫力，再加上快速诊断和有效疗法的普及，与严重急性呼吸系统综合征冠状病毒 2 型相关的发病率和死亡率已显著下降。

2. 流感、呼吸道合胞病毒、人偏肺病毒、副流感病毒和其他呼吸道病毒的院内传播和集群事件以意想不到的频率发生。

3. 无论医疗机构的口罩政策如何，工作人员都会经常接触到呼吸道病毒，因为他们中的大多数人在不工作时不再佩戴口罩。因此，没有必要强迫他们在病人护理时间之外佩戴口罩。

4. A higher viral infection rate in the population increases the likelihood that a health care provider, visitor, or patient may contract the virus and spread it to another patient.

5. By implementing a system that applies masks to all patients during periods of high viral activity and to the most susceptible individuals all year round, they can better safeguard their patients from the full spectrum of nosocomial respiratory viral infections.

Text B

After Reading Activities:

Reading Comprehension

Decide whether the following statements are true (T) or false (F) according to the text.

1. F 2. F 3. T 4. T 5. T

Words and Phrases

Match each English phrase in Column A with its Chinese version in Column B.

1. H 2. D 3. F 4. A 5. G 6. B 7. C 8. E

Translation

Public-health officials have long sought a vaccine against malaria, which infects up to 600 million people a year and kills 400,000, mostly children. In 2021, there was dramatic progress on this front. In a study of 450 children, researchers reported that a new malaria vaccine, called R21, is 77% effective. The sample group for the study was comparatively small, though, and more research is needed. Investigators working for an international team, including the University of Oxford, plan to follow the initial sample group for longer and will conduct other trials in countries where malaria is active year-round.

Critical Thinking

One policy enacted by the Chinese government aiming to guarantee public health is the "Healthy China 2030" initiative. This policy was introduced in 2016 with the goal of improving the overall health of the Chinese population and building a more robust health care system.

The "Healthy China 2030" initiative focuses on several key areas:

1. Health promotion and disease prevention: The policy emphasizes the importance of health education and the promotion of healthy lifestyles to prevent chronic diseases, such as cardiovascular diseases, diabetes, cancer, and respiratory diseases. It encourages the

adoption of healthier diets, regular physical activity, and the reduction of tobacco and alcohol consumption.

2. Health service capacity building: The initiative aims to improve the quality and accessibility of health care services. This includes enhancing primary health care services, developing a tiered medical system, and promoting the use of traditional Chinese medicine alongside Western medicine.

3. Health insurance coverage: The policy seeks to expand and improve the coverage of health insurance, ensuring that all citizens have access to essential medical services without facing financial burdens.

4. Public health and safety: The initiative focuses on strengthening the public health system, improving infectious disease control, and enhancing the capacity for emergency response and disaster management.

5. Health industry development: The policy supports the growth of the health industry, including pharmaceuticals, medical devices, and health-related services, to create a more diverse and competitive market.

6. Health governance: The initiative emphasizes the importance of strengthening health governance, including regulatory oversight, monitoring and evaluation systems, and the establishment of a national health information platform.

How this policy works:

—Multi-sectoral collaboration: The "Healthy China 2030" initiative involves collaboration between various government departments, including health, finance, education, and agriculture, to ensure a comprehensive approach to public health.

—Policy implementation: The government has developed detailed action plans and targets for each area of focus within the initiative. These are implemented through legislation, regulations, and specific programs.

—Investment in health care infrastructure: The government has increased funding for health care infrastructure, including the construction of new hospitals, clinics, and research facilities.

—Public awareness and education: There is a strong emphasis on public education campaigns to raise awareness about healthy lifestyles and the importance of preventive health care.

—Performance monitoring: The progress of the initiative is monitored through regular evaluations and assessments, ensuring that goals are met and adjustments can be made where necessary.

Overall, the "Healthy China 2030" initiative is a comprehensive strategy that aims to improve the health of the Chinese population through a combination of health promotion, service enhancement, insurance expansion, and industry development. By focusing on both individual behavior and systemic improvements, the policy seeks to create a healthier society and a more resilient health care system.

Part III   Apply Medical English

Practical Activity

Patient: What do you think? Am I OK?

Doctor: Let me check your blood pressure. Please roll up your sleeve and rest your arm on the table. Okay, now I'm going to inflate the cuff around your upper arm. Just relax and stay still.

Patient: Alright, doctor.

Doctor: Your blood pressure is a bit high. It's 150 over 90. You have hypertension. We need to monitor it regularly and make some lifestyle changes.

Patient: What should I do to control my blood pressure?

Doctor: Firstly, you need to maintain a healthy weight by eating a balanced diet and exercising regularly. Secondly, reduce the amount of salt in your diet, as excessive salt consumption can lead to an increase in blood pressure. Thirdly, limit your alcohol intake and quit smoking if you smoke. Fourthly, manage your stress levels through relaxation techniques such as meditation or yoga. Finally, take any prescribed medication as directed by your health care provider.

Patient: Will these changes be enough to lower my blood pressure?

Doctor: These lifestyle modifications can help lower your blood pressure significantly. However, it's important to follow up with regular check-ups and monitoring. If necessary, we may prescribe medication to help control your blood pressure.

Patient: Thank you, doctor. I will start making these changes right away.

Doctor: You're welcome. Remember, managing hypertension requires a commitment to long-term lifestyle changes. Don't hesitate to reach out if you have any concerns or questions.

B. Practical Unit Project (略)

Unit 2   Keys to Exercises and Audio Scripts

Part I   View the Medical World

1. D   2. B   3. C   4. A   5. C

Script

In 1965, 17-year-old high school student, Randy Gardner stayed awake for 264 hours. That's 11 days to see how he'd cope without sleep.

On the second day, his eyes stopped focusing. Next, he lost the ability to identify objects by touch. By day three, Gardner was moody and uncoordinated.

At the end of the experiment, he was struggling to concentrate, had trouble with short-term memory, became paranoid, and started hallucinating. Although Gardner recovered without long-term psychological or physical damage, for others, losing shuteye can result in hormonal imbalance, illness, and, in extreme cases, death.

We're only beginning to understand why we sleep to begin with, but we do know it's essential. Adults need seven to eight hours of sleep a night, and adolescents need about ten. We grow sleepy due to signals from our body telling our brain we are tired, and signals from the environment telling us it's dark outside.

The rise in sleep-inducing chemicals, like adenosine and melatonin, send us into a light doze that grows deeper, making our breathing and heart rate slow down and our muscles relax. This non-REM sleep is when DNA is repaired and our bodies replenish themselves for the day ahead.

In the United States, it's estimated that 30% of adults and 66% of adolescents are regularly sleep-deprived. This isn't just a minor inconvenience. Staying awake can cause serious bodily harm. When we lose sleep, learning, memory, mood, and reaction time are affected. Sleeplessness may also cause inflammation, hallucinations, high blood pressure, and it's even been linked to diabetes and obesity.

In 2014, a devoted soccer fan died after staying awake for 48 hours to watch the World Cup. While his untimely death was due to a stroke, studies show that chronically sleeping fewer than six hours a night increases stroke risk by four and half times compared to those getting a consistent seven to eight hours of shuteye.

For a handful of people on the planet who carry a rare inherited genetic mutation, sleeplessness is a daily reality. This condition, known as Fatal Familial Insomnia, places the body in a nightmarish state of wakefulness, forbidding it from entering the sanctuary of sleep. Within months or years, this progressively worsening condition leads to dementia and death.

How can sleep deprivation cause such immense suffering? Scientists think the answer lies with the accumulation of waste products in the brain. During our waking hours, our cells are busy using up our day's energy sources, which get broken down into various byproducts, including adenosine. As adenosine builds up, it increases the urge to sleep, also known as sleep pressure.

In fact, caffeine works by blocking adenosine's receptor pathways. Other waste products also build up in the brain, and if they're not cleared away, they collectively overload the brain and are thought to lead to the many negative symptoms of sleep deprivation.

So, what's happening in our brain when we sleep to prevent this? Scientists found something called the glymphatic system, a clean-up mechanism that removes this buildup and is much more active when we're asleep. It works by using cerebrospinal fluid to flush away toxic byproducts that accumulate between cells. Lymphatic vessels, which serve as pathways for immune cells, have recently been discovered in the brain, and they may also play a role in clearing out the brain's daily waste products.

While scientists continue exploring the restorative mechanisms behind sleep, we can be sure that slipping into slumber is a necessity if we want to maintain our health and our sanity.

Part II　Read to Explore Medical Knowledge

Text A

After Reading Activities:

Reading Comprehension

Ⅰ. Answer the following questions.

1. Given the global concern over population ageing, it is imperative to identify interventions that are both accessible and affordable in order to promote healthy ageing. Adopting a healthy lifestyle will likely be crucial.

2. Although excessive physical activity might bring more harms than benefits for people older than 60 years, this study suggested that 7. 5 to less than 15 MET hours per week of any activity is sufficient to reduce mortality risks, with racquet sports and running being the most

beneficial.

3. Living with other people predicted slower global cognitive, memory, and language decline than living alone, and weekly interactions with family and friends and weekly community group engagement predicted slower memory decline than no interactions and no engagement. These findings emphasize the importance of social connections for the mental health of people older than 60 years, and might encourage family members and the community to offer more group activities for older members.

4. The six healthy lifestyle factors are what people eat, how often they exercise, how active they are socially and cognitively, whether they smoke or not, and whether they drink alcohol or not.

5. A longer life expectancy is just one of the goals of good ageing; other objectives include better mental and physical health as well as overall well-being for those over the age of 60.

II. Work in groups to complete the following chart according to the structure of the text.

Introduction and thesis statement: (para. 1)

accessible, crucial

Accessible and affordable interventions and healthy lifestyle choices: (paras. 2-6)

chronic disease, appropriate hydration, mortality risks, interactions, neurocognitive

Conclusion: (para. 7)

processes

Words and Phrases

I. Translate the following medical terms into Chinese or English.

1. 血清钠水平　　　　5. hydration status

2. 神经认知健康　　　6. dose-response

3. 抗炎反应　　　　　7. systolic and diastolic blood pressure

4. 代谢当量　　　　　8. cardiometabolic risk factor

II. Fill in the blanks with the words or phrases given below. Change the form if necessary.

1. concentration

2. Favorable

3. Expenditure

4. induced

5. prospect

Sentence Translation

1. 与对照组的参与者相比，热量限制饮食组的参与者在低密度脂蛋白胆固醇、总胆固醇与高密度脂蛋白胆固醇的比率以及收缩压和舒张压等常规心脏代谢风险因素上都持续显著降低。

2. 正常血清钠水平高(142 至<146 mmol/l)的中年人(45~66 岁)患心力衰竭、痴呆症、慢性肺病和中风等慢性疾病的风险增加了 39%。

3. 限制卡路里摄入量是维持体内平衡的一种方法，而增加能量消耗(通过运动等方式)则是保持能量水平稳定的另一种方法。

4. Global cognitive, memory, and language decline was slowed by living with others rather than alone, and memory decline was slowed by engaging with community groups once a week and by interacting with family and friends once a week.

5. The need to comprehend the processes of ageing and create treatments to avoid or postpone the commencement of age-related illnesses is of increasingly great importance and urgency due to the increase in the population of individuals aged over 60.

Text B

After Reading Activities：

Reading Comprehension

Decide whether the following statements are true (T) or false (F) according to the text.

1. F   2. F   3. F   4. T   5. T

Match each English phrase in Column A with its Chinese version in Column B.

1. H   2. D   3. F   4. A   5. G   6. B   7. C   8. E

Translation

Healthy eating doesn't have to be overly complicated. If you feel overwhelmed by all the conflicting nutrition and diet advice out there, you're not alone. It seems that for every expert who tells you a certain food is good for you; you'll find another saying exactly the opposite. The truth is that while some specific foods or nutrients have been shown to have a beneficial effect on mood, it's your overall dietary pattern that is most important. The cornerstone of a healthy diet should be to replace processed food with real food whenever possible. Eating food that is as close as possible to the way nature made it can make a huge difference to the way you think, look, and feel.

Critical Thinking（略）

Part III　Apply Medical English

Practical Activity

Doctor: Good morning! How are you feeling today?

Patient (child): Hi, doctor. I'm not feeling so good. My throat hurts, and I have a fever.

Doctor: I'm sorry to hear that. Let's see if we can figure out what's going on. Have you been coughing or having trouble breathing?

Patient: Yeah, I've been coughing a lot, and it's hard to breathe sometimes.

Doctor: Okay, I see. Have you noticed any other symptoms, like a runny nose or a headache?

Patient: Yeah, my nose has been running, and my head hurts too.

Doctor: Alright, thank you for letting me know. Now, I'm going to take a look at your throat and listen to your chest, okay?

Patient: Okay.

[The doctor examines the child's throat and listens to their chest with a stethoscope.]

Doctor: It looks like you have a sore throat and your chest sounds a bit congested. Based on your symptoms, it's possible that you have a respiratory infection, like the common cold or the flu.

Patient: Oh no, does that mean I have to get a shot?

Doctor: Not necessarily. Most respiratory infections are caused by viruses, so antibiotics won't help. However, I may recommend some treatments to help you feel better, like getting plenty of rest, drinking fluids, and taking over-the-counter pain relievers for your fever and sore throat.

Patient: Okay, I can do that. Will I feel better soon?

Doctor: With some rest and TLC, you should start feeling better in a few days. But if your symptoms get worse or you have trouble breathing, it's important to let me know right away, okay?

Patient: Alright, I will. Thank you, doctor.

Doctor: You're welcome. Take care, and I'll see you again soon to check on your progress.

[The doctor and patient exchange smiles before the patient leaves the room.]

B. Practical Unit Project

Dear Su Shi,

I hope this letter finds you well. I wanted to take a moment to share some thoughts and suggestions regarding maintaining a healthy lifestyle, particularly in terms of diet and alcohol consumption.

Firstly, let's discuss diet. It's essential to prioritize whole, nutrient-rich foods in your daily meals. Aim to include plenty of fruits, vegetables, whole grains, lean proteins, and healthy fats in your diet. These foods provide essential vitamins, minerals, and antioxidants that support overall health and well-being.

Additionally, be mindful of portion sizes and practice moderation when indulging in less nutritious foods or treats. Remember that balance is the key, and it's okay to enjoy your favorite foods in moderation while prioritizing nutrient-dense options for the majority of your meals.

When it comes to alcohol consumption, moderation is also crucial. While enjoying a drink occasionally can be a part of a healthy lifestyle, excessive alcohol intake can have negative effects on your health, including increased risk of liver disease, heart problems, and mental health issues.

Consider setting limits on how much alcohol you consume and stick to them. Opt for lower-alcohol options, alternate alcoholic drinks with water or non-alcoholic beverages, and be mindful of the size of your drinks. Prioritize quality over quantity and savor each sip mindfully.

In addition to diet and alcohol consumption, there are several other aspects of a healthy lifestyle to consider. Regular physical activity is essential for maintaining overall health and well-being. Aim for at least 150 minutes of moderate-intensity aerobic activity or 75 minutes of vigorous-intensity activity per week, as recommended by health guidelines.

Prioritize sleep by aiming for 7-9 hours of quality sleep each night and establishing a regular sleep schedule. Create a relaxing bedtime routine and ensure your sleep environment is comfortable and conducive to restful sleep.

Lastly, don't forget to prioritize stress management and self-care. Practice relaxation techniques such as deep breathing, mindfulness meditation, or yoga to reduce stress and promote mental well-being. Take time for activities you enjoy, spend time outdoors in nature, and nurture your relationships with friends and family.

Overall, maintaining a healthy lifestyle is about finding balance, making mindful choices, and prioritizing self-care. By incorporating these suggestions into your daily routine, you can support your overall health and well-being and enjoy a fulfilling and vibrant life.

Wishing you health and happiness,

[Your Name]

Unit 3　Keys to Exercises and Audio Scripts

Part I　View the Medical World

1. A　2. C　3. B　4. D　5. D

Script

　　Today we're going to talk about the modern health care system in the United States and get a history in timeline of how we got to where we are today. In 1901, the American Medical Association becomes a National Organization. Membership goes from about 8,000 physicians in 1900 to 70,000 in 1910. This is the beginning of organized medicine. Doctors are no longer expected to provide free services to all hospital patients. The Depression in the 1930s changes the country's priorities to a greater emphasis on unemployment insurance and old-age benefits. The Social Security Act is passed but doesn't even mention health insurance. In the 1940s, penicillin becomes widely used and has a dramatic effect on the leading cause of death at the time—infection. During the Second World War, wage and price controls are placed on American employers. To compete for workers, companies begin to offer health benefits, giving rise to the employer-based system we have in place today. President Roosevelt asked Congress for an economic Bill of Rights, including the right to adequate medical care. By the 1950s, more medications are available to treat a range of diseases, including infections, glaucoma, and arthritis. New vaccines become available that prevent dreaded childhood diseases like polio. The first successful organ transplant is performed and the price of hospital care doubles because of all of the new services. In the early 1960s, those outside the workplace, especially the elderly, have difficulty affording insurance. President Lyndon Johnson signs Medicare and Medicaid into law. The number of doctors calling themselves specialists grows from 55% in 1960 to 69% by the end of the decade. By the 1970s, health care costs are escalating rapidly, partially due to the higher than predicted Medicare costs along with rapidly rising inflation. People are living longer with the greater use of technology, more medication and a growing list of expensive cutting-edge treatments. People start to question if the American medical system can sustain itself with the rising costs. In the 80s, corporations begin to integrate the hospital system, previously a decentralized structure. Overall, there's a shift towards privatization and corporatization of health care. By the 1990s, health care costs rise at double the rate of inflation. In the 2000s, health care costs continue to rise and Medicare is viewed by most experts as unsustainable for the coming baby boomer population. Premiums going up by double digits each year, along with the ageing of the workforce, lead many to believe that health insurance through your employer can't last. Direct-to-consumer advertising for pharmaceuticals and medical devices begin to engage the consumer in the process. The internet begins to put quality medical information in front of consumers both from news sources like WebMD, and trusted Centers of Excellence like the Mayo Clinic and others. By 2010, Facebook, Twitter, YouTube, and other social networking sites continue to revolutionize communication. Consumers go online to learn about everything, including their health. The passage of the Affordable Care Act makes major changes to the future of care, putting more emphasis on prevention and detection. In 2012, a Silicon Valley doctor launches Step One Health and easy connection to new health care. Step One Health is a digital starting line that allows consumers to be proactive informed and in charge of their health care decisions. Step One Health combines easy access to early detection and prevention with a community of connected people changing the health care experience.

Part II   Read to Explore Medical Knowledge

Text A

After Reading Activities:

Reading Comprehension

I. Answer the following questions.

1. Because it failed to cope with such problems as the poor health and rather high mortality of the population, the relative underinvestment in primary care, the administrative inefficiency of the system, and the pervasive disparities in the delivery of care.

2. The key strategies for improving the health of a country's population through health care are to promote timely access to preventive, acute, and chronic care and to deliver evidence-based and appropriate care services.

3. Yes. The United States performs on equal or even better than other nations in a number of patient-centered care processes, and on disease-specific outcomes for acute myocardial infarction, ischemic stroke, colon cancer, and breast cancer.

4. Lack of access to health care is the first problem the American health care system has to deal with. The second problem is that, in comparison to other nations, the United States invests

very little in primary care. The third problem is the American health care system's administrative inefficiencies. The fourth problem is the widespread existence of inequalities in health care delivery in the United States.

5. Millions of people have gained affordable insurance coverage and access to care under the ACA, and more could gain coverage through further Medicaid expansion and stabilization of individual insurance markets. Moreover, the ACA strengthened the Centers for Medicare and Medicaid Services' ability to push for payment reforms that support primary care.

II. Work in groups to complete the following chart according to the structure of the text.

What is the problem: (paras. 1-2)

placed the United States' health care system worst,

falls short of health care systems,

Causes of the problem: (paras. 3-8)

the cost of care and its affordability for individuals,

the administrative burden (or hassle) that people confront as they obtain and receive care,

and disparities or inequities in the delivery of care based on income, educational attainment, race or ethnic background, or other nonclinical personal characteristics

lack of access to health care is the first problem the American health care system has to deal with,

the second problem is, in comparison to other nations, the underinvestment in primary care in the United States.

the third problem is the American health care system's administrative inefficiencies,

the fourth problem is the pervasiveness in the United States of disparities in the delivery of care.

Solutions to the problems: (paras. 9-10)

launching coordinated efforts to address each of these problems,

universal and sufficient health insurance coverage,

primary care,

administrative costs,

income-related gaps.

Conclusion: (para. 11)

first,

the health of its citizens,

new laws,

renewed commitments

Words and Phrases

I. Translate the following medical terms into Chinese or English.

1. 医疗保险覆盖面   5. myocardial infarction

2. 延迟诊断   6. ischemic stroke

3. 初级护理   7. colon cancer

4. 专科护理   8. preventive care

II. Fill in the blanks with the words or phrases given below. Change the form if necessary.

1. chronic   4. acute

2. mortality   5. pervasive

3. preventive

Sentence Translation

1. 一个高效的医疗保障系统的目的就在于提供保障，提高个体及整个国家人口的健康水平。

2. 通过医疗保障来提高整个国家人口的健康水平包括以下策略：提供及时的预防性、急性和慢性护理以及循证的、适当的医疗服务。

3. 可承担的和全面的医疗保险是根本。如果人们没有医保，一些人就会推迟就医，其中一些人会出现严重的健康问题，甚至有一些人会面临死亡。

4. Conversely, since 2004, assessments published by the Commonwealth Fund have repeatedly placed the United States' health care system worst among high-income nations, even though our country spends a lot more money on health care than these other nations.

5. Clinicians and their staff spend countless hours completing documentation to prove that insurance coverage is active, that benefits and services are covered, that services were delivered, and that payment or reimbursement occurred.

Text B

After Reading Activities：

Reading Comprehension

Decide whether the following statements are true (T) or false (F) according to the text.

1. T   2. F   3. F   4. T   5. F

Match each English phrase in Column A with its Chinese version in Column B.

1. B   2. D   3. H   4. G   5. F   6. A   7. E   8. C

Translation

At present, there are three kinds of medical insurance policies in China: one is the urban employee insurance system established in 1998; the other two are the new rural cooperative medical system established in 2003, and the urban residents medical system established in 2007. Among them, the latter two are highly subsidized by the government, while the policy for the urban employed, paid by employees and their employers, has the best reimbursement rate.

Critical Thinking

Here's a comparison of the health care systems between China and the U. S. based on the information from our texts:

1. Health Care Coverage:

—China: The Chinese health care system aims to provide universal coverage to all citizens. It is primarily funded through government subsidies, social insurance, and out-of-pocket payments. The New Rural Cooperative Medical Scheme (NCMS) covers rural residents, while the Urban Employee Basic Medical Insurance (UEBMI) and Urban Resident Basic Medical Insurance (URBMI) cover urban workers and residents, respectively.

—U.S. : The U.S. has a mixed health care system with both public and private insurance options. Medicare and Medicaid provide coverage for older adults, people with disabilities, and low-income individuals and families. However, many Americans obtain health insurance through their employers or purchase it individually in the private market. A significant portion of the population remains uninsured or underinsured.

2. Health Care Delivery:

—China: The Chinese health care system includes a mix of public hospitals, private hospitals, and clinics. Public hospitals are the dominant providers and are generally more affordable than private facilities. The government heavily regulates the prices of medical services and drugs to keep costs down.

—U.S. : The U.S. has a diverse health care delivery system with a mix of public and private hospitals, clinics, and other health care facilities. Private practice is common, and there is a wide range of pricing for medical services and drugs.

3. Health Care Financing:

—China: The Chinese government plays a significant role in financing the health care system through taxes and social insurance contributions. Out-of-pocket expenses are also required for certain services, but the government caps these fees to prevent excessive costs for patients.

—U.S. : Health care financing in the U.S. is complex, involving private insurance companies, government programs, and out-of-pocket payments by individuals. The high cost of health care in the U.S. is a significant issue, with administrative expenses and drug prices contributing to the overall expense.

4. Access to Care:

—China: Despite efforts to provide universal coverage, access to care can vary across different regions of China, with urban areas typically having better resources than rural ones. However, the government is working to improve infrastructure and increase the number of health care professionals, especially in less developed areas.

—U.S. : Access to care in the U.S. is influenced by multiple factors, including insurance status, geographic location, and availability of health care providers. Rural areas often face challenges in accessing specialized care, and there are disparities in health outcomes among different socioeconomic groups.

5. Quality of Care:

—China: The Chinese government has made strides in improving the quality of care, investing in medical education and training for health care professionals. However, there are still concerns about the quality of care in some areas, particularly in overcrowded hospitals and remote regions.

—U.S. : The U.S. is known for having some of the world's best medical facilities and highly skilled medical professionals. However, the quality of care can vary significantly, with disparities seen among different racial and socioeconomic groups.

6. Preventive Care and Public Health:

—China: The Chinese government emphasizes preventive care and public health initiatives, such as vaccination programs and campaigns against tobacco use. There is also a focus on traditional Chinese medicine and integrating it into the mainstream health care system.

—U.S. : The U.S. has a strong history of public health initiatives and invests in preventive care measures. However, funding for public health programs can be politically contentious, and there are ongoing debates about the effectiveness and prioritization of various preventive strategies.

In summary, while both China and the U.S. aim to provide comprehensive health care to their citizens, they approach this goal through different systems with varying degrees of government involvement, coverage, and access to care. The Chinese system leans more towards government control and universal coverage, while the U.S. system is more fragmented and relies more heavily on private insurance and individual responsibility.

Part III   Apply Medical English

Practical Activity

Nurse: Hello! Welcome to our clinic. How can I assist you today?

Patient: Hi! I'm here to fill out the registration form.

Nurse: Great! Let's start with your name. What is your full name?

Patient: My name is John Smith.

Nurse: Thank you, John Smith. Can you please provide me with your date of birth?

Patient: Sure, my date of birth is January 15, 1990.

Nurse: Thank you. Now, let's move on to your address. Could you please provide me with your Chinese address as well as your home country address?

Patient: My Chinese address is 328 Renmin Road, Shanghai, China, and my home country address is 123 Main Street, New York, United States.

Nurse: Perfect. Now, could you please tell me your nationality?

Patient: I'm an American citizen.

Nurse: Got it. And do you have a passport number that I can include in your records?

Patient: Yes, my passport number is G123456789.

Nurse: Thank you. Lastly, could you please provide me with your telephone number and medical insurance number?

Patient: Sure, my telephone number is +86-13800138000, and my medical insurance number is M123456.

Nurse: Wonderful! All the information has been recorded. Is there anything else I can help you with?

Patient: No, that's all for now. Thank you for your assistance!

Nurse: You're welcome! If you have any further questions or need any additional help, feel free to ask. Take care!

Patient: Thank you! Take care too!

B. Practical Unit Project (略)

Unit 4 Keys to Exercises and Audio Scripts

Part I View the Medical World

1. B   2. A   3. C   4. D   5. C

Script

Today's topic is acupuncture: what you need to know. Holistic medical procedures might seem useless or scary to those with no knowledge of them. This goes for acupuncture as well. After all, how can having yourself being pricked by dozens of needles at the same time be helpful and not just painful? However, the one aspect you cannot ignore about acupuncture is that the procedure has been around 2500 years, and people have sworn by its benefits all those years. It is said to work miracles and has been attributed to helping with conditions ranging from depression to morning sickness. It is supposed to play a big role in improving quality of life, but what is it exactly and how does it work? Let's look at acupuncture in detail.

What is it? Acupuncture is a technique coming from ancient China that involves pricking the skin with needles to trigger specific points on it. The traditional philosophy behind it leans towards the metaphysical. The ancient Chinese believed that the human body had a network of life force in it, known as qi. They aim to heal the body by manipulating this qi with the aid of needles. Nowadays acupuncture is supported by modern science as a means to stimulate the body's nervous system by pricking the body in certain areas. Acupuncture gives the brain an idea of where to focus. It is believed to work by essentially stimulating the brain's activity towards the parts of the body that require its attention.

What does it do? You might want to try out acupuncture for several reasons. It is, after all, supposed to help with countless conditions, although there is no medical proof to support it. Acupuncture is believed to help with: 1. strokes, 2. allergies, 3. anxiety and depression, 4. hypertension, 5. insomnia, 6. osteoarthritis, 7. chronic pain in different parts of the body, 8. menstrual cramps, 9. PMS, 10. migraines, 11. sprains, 12. morning sickness. Furthermore, some people even claim that the procedure can help with the treatment of multiple sclerosis and cancer although there is limited backing for this.

How to add it to your life? It is quite easy to find an acupuncturist and the sessions are relatively inexpensive. Sessions can last from 30 to 90 minutes, just a small portion of your day. However, you do not need a session every day. In fact, even once a week might be more than you need. Of course, everyone responds to the treatment differently. So, it might be a while before you feel its effects, be patient with it and do not try to be hasty. If there is no acupuncturist in your city, or you cannot get a session, do not try it by yourself ever. It is a delicate procedure and needs to be carried out by trained hands. It is much better to plan a trip to a nearby city with one rather than taking such a big risk. Thank you for watching our video, and please do not forget to like and share the video.

Part II Read to Explore Medical Knowledge

Text A

After Reading Activities:

Reading Comprehension

I. Answer the following questions.

1. Qi travels through the body via particular channels known as meridians or vessels. Health is preserved as long as this energy is allowed to freely move through the meridians; but, as soon as this energy flow is obstructed, the system becomes unstable, leading to discomfort and dysfunction.

2. Acupuncture causes the release of endorphins from the brain. Endorphins are responsible for the relaxation and mood-lifting experiences people have during these activities. As well, endorphins are also effective at reducing levels of pain.

3. Pain usually occurs when a disease or injury is causing poor blood flow or impaired nerve transmission. Depending on the underlying causes, a healthy body will react differently to heal the issues and reduce discomfort.

4. Food, oxygen, hormones, medicine, and substances that stave off infection and aid in healing are all found in your blood. Longevity and optimal health are dependent on the blood traveling to the right places in your body and staying there. The majority of diseases and injuries can manifest if these essential compounds are not delivered to their intended location.

5. Acupuncture serves as a way of promoting preventive care and symptom management for children to harmonize traditional Western medicine and Traditional Chinese.

II. Work in groups to complete the following chart according to the structure of the text.

The introduction (paras. 1-2)

Traditional Chinese Medicine, cornerstone

How does Acupuncture work (para. 3)

meridians, pain and dysfunction, reprogram, restore, free up

Six functions of Acupuncture: (paras. 4-15)

1. neurochemicals, hormones   4. knee arthritis

2. blood   5. fertility

3. severe heart failure   6. chronic pain

Words and Phrases

I. Translate the following medical terms into Chinese or English.

1. 引发好转反应   5. deficient pattern

2. 止痛   6. excess pattern

3. 抗炎蛋白   7. menstrual pain

4. 儿科针灸   8. blood clot

II. Fill in the blanks with the words or phrases given below. Change the form if necessary.

1. modulate   4. stagnation

2. fertility   5. regimen

3. serve to

Sentence Translation

1. 鉴于目前针刺疗法研究的大力发展，加上各家庭积极地参与支持和产生很少的副作用，针刺疗法可以作为一种在提高儿童预防保健和症状管理的方法来协调传统西医和传统中医。

2. 只要身体里的气沿着经络自由畅通行走，我们就能保持身体健康。

3. 在同一批接受试管婴儿手术的患者中，伴有针刺疗法辅助的患者约有 40% 已经成功怀孕了，相比之下，没有接受针刺疗法辅助的患者只有 26% 的成功率。

4. Acupuncture stimulates specific meridians, which then helps to reprogram and restore normal function.

5. It is believed that this energy travels through the body via particular channels known as

meridians or vessels. Health is preserved as long as this energy is allowed to freely move through the meridians; but, as soon as this energy flow is obstructed, the system becomes unstable, leading to discomfort and dysfunction.

Text B

After Reading Activities:

Reading Comprehension

Decide whether the following statements are true (T) or false (F) according to the text.

1. T   2. T   3. F   4. T   5. F

Match each English phrase in Column A with its Chinese version in Column B.

1. C   2. G   3. D   4. F   5. A   6. B   7. H   8. E

Translation

TCM practitioners believe that all the different organs and systems within the body form an interconnected, organic whole. Each part of this whole can be described as either yin or yang. If the flow of qi is blocked or the blood is stagnant, imbalances in a person's yin and yang can result. According to Traditional Chinese Medicine, these imbalances can lead to health problems, so many TCM therapies focus on restoring this balance. When making a diagnosis, TCM doctors use various methods including inquiry, inspection, palpation, olfaction (smelling) and auscultation (listening). It's also common for TCM doctors to take patients' pulse and examine their tongues before deciding on a course of treatment.

Critical Thinking

As a student of medicine, I believe that both Traditional Chinese Medicine (TCM) and Western medicine have their strengths and limitations, and their collaboration holds great promise for improving patient care in the future.

TCM offers a holistic approach to health and well-being, focusing on restoring balance and harmony within the body. It has a long history of use in treating various ailments and can be particularly effective for chronic conditions like heart disease, as well as for promoting overall wellness. TCM modalities such as acupuncture, herbal medicine, and therapeutic exercises offer complementary options for patients seeking alternative or adjunctive treatments.

On the other hand, Western medicine is highly evidence-based and relies on rigorous scientific research to develop diagnostic and treatment approaches. It excels in acute care, surgical interventions, and the management of infectious diseases through techniques such as antibiotics and vaccinations. Western medicine also utilizes advanced technologies such as imaging studies and laboratory tests for precise diagnosis and monitoring of disease progression.

In terms of collaboration, I believe there's immense potential for TCM and Western medicine to work synergistically. By integrating the strengths of both systems, health care providers can offer patients a more comprehensive and personalized approach to treatment. For example, combining acupuncture or herbal remedies with conventional therapies for heart disease may enhance outcomes and improve quality of life for patients.

However, it's essential to approach collaboration with caution and respect for each system's principles and practices. This includes fostering interdisciplinary communication, sharing knowledge and expertise, and conducting rigorous research to evaluate the safety and efficacy of integrated approaches.

Ultimately, the goal should be to provide patients with the best possible care, drawing on the strengths of both TCM and Western medicine while recognizing the unique needs and preferences of individual patients. By embracing collaboration and open-mindedness, we can harness the full potential of both systems to advance health care and improve patient outcomes.

Part III   Apply Medical English

Practical Activity

Doctor: Good afternoon, how can I assist you today?

Patient: Hello doctor, I've been experiencing some digestive issues lately, including bloating and occasional stomach discomfort. I've heard about herbal medicine and was wondering if it could help alleviate my symptoms.

Doctor: I'm sorry to hear that you've been dealing with digestive issues. Herbal medicine can indeed offer natural remedies that may help address your symptoms. Before we proceed, could you please tell me more about your symptoms and any factors that may have triggered them?

Patient: Of course. The bloating and discomfort tend to occur after meals, especially when I eat certain foods like dairy or spicy dishes. I've also noticed some irregularity in my bowel movements.

Doctor: I see. Let me take a moment to observe your overall appearance and demeanor. Could you please extend your arm so I can feel your pulse?

[*The doctor observes the patient's complexion, posture, and general appearance, as well as the condition of the patient's tongue.*]

Doctor: Based on what I've observed, your complexion appears slightly pale, which can be indicative of deficient energy or blood circulation. Your tongue also shows signs of slight coating and moisture, indicating potential internal imbalances.

Patient: That's interesting. What does that mean for my treatment?

Doctor: These observations, along with the information you've provided about your symptoms, suggest that there may be underlying imbalances in your digestive system, which herbal medicine can help address. Now, if you don't mind, I'd like to feel your pulse to further assess your condition.

[*The doctor takes the patient's pulse at various points on the wrist and notes the strength, rhythm, and quality of the pulse.*]

Doctor: Your pulse feels slightly weak and irregular, particularly in the positions corresponding to the spleen and stomach meridians. This further supports the possibility of digestive imbalances contributing to your symptoms.

Patient: I see. So, how does herbal medicine work, and what can I expect during the treatment?

Doctor: Herbal medicine involves using natural plant-based remedies to support the body's healing process and restore balance. I'll prescribe a customized herbal formula tailored to address your specific symptoms and underlying imbalances. You can expect to take the herbal remedies as directed, typically in the form of teas, capsules, or powders, and we'll monitor your progress over time to adjust the treatment as needed.

Patient: That sounds like it could be helpful for my condition. When can we start the herbal treatment?

Doctor: Excellent! Let's go ahead and discuss your personalized herbal formula, and I'll provide you with detailed instructions on how to take it. In the meantime, I'll also offer you some dietary and lifestyle recommendations to complement the herbal treatment and optimize your digestive health.

Patient: Thank you so much, doctor. I appreciate your thorough assessment and guidance.

B. Practical Unit Project (略)

Unit 5   Keys to Exercises and Audio Scripts

Part I   View the Medical World

1. C   2. A   3. D   4. B   5. B

Script

Clinical depression is different. It's a medical disorder, and it won't go away just because you want it to. It lingers for at least two consecutive weeks, and significantly interferes with one's ability to work, play or love. Depression can have a lot of different symptoms: a low mood, loss of interest in things you'd normally enjoy, changes in appetite, feeling worthless or excessively guilty, sleeping either too much or too little, poor concentration, restlessness or slowness, loss of energy or recurrent thoughts of suicide. If you have at least five of those symptoms, according to psychiatric guidelines, you qualify for a diagnosis of depression. And it's not just behavioral symptoms. Depression has physical manifestations inside the brain. First of all, there are changes that could be seen with the naked eye and X-ray vision. These include smaller frontal lobes and hippocampal volumes. On a more micro scale, depression is associated with a few things: the abnormal transmission or depletion of certain neurotransmitters, especially serotonin, norepinephrine and dopamine, blunted circadian rhythms, or specific changes in the REM and slow-wave parts of your sleep cycle, and hormone abnormalities, such as high cortisol and deregulation of thyroid hormones. But neuroscientists still don't have a complete picture of what causes depression. It seems to have to do with a complex interaction between genes and environment, but we don't have a diagnostic tool that can accurately predict where or when it will show up. And because depression symptoms are intangible, it's hard to know who might look fine but is actually struggling. According to the National Institute of Mental Health, it takes the average person suffering with a mental illness over ten years to ask for help.

Part II   Read to Explore Medical Knowledge

Text A

After Reading Activities:

Reading Comprehension

I. Answer the following questions.

1. Cognitive behavioral therapy (CBT), antidepressant medications, psychodynamic therapy, exercise, transcranial magnetic stimulation, electroconvulsive therapy.

2. Neither of these treatments is more effective than the other.

3. Psychotherapies can span months and include several hour-long sessions, which is too much for many individuals. Some people might not be able to afford the treatment they need because they do not have access to mental health professionals. Some people might prefer to take medication at home rather than disclose personal information in a medical setting.

4. There are other treatment options include: exercise, transcranial magnetic stimulation and electroconvulsive therapy.

5. As the ACP guidelines recommend, clinicians should talk with patients about "treatment effects, adverse effect profiles, cost, accessibility, and preferences with the patient" while treating depression.

II. Work in groups to complete the following chart according to the structure of the text.

The problem both patients and doctors facing: (paras. 1-3)

16 million Americans, embarking on, various forms of medical treatment

The effectiveness of treatments for depression: (paras. 4-11)

psychotherapies, antidepressants, the efficacy of combining these therapies, "similarly effective treatments"

Doctors' and patients' choice for treating depression and the reasons behind: (paras. 12-17)

antidepressants, other treatments, The utilization of antidepressants, the utilization of psychotherapy, too much for many individuals, mental health professionals, disclose personal information in a medical setting

Other treatment options in addition to therapy and medication: (paras. 18-21)

exercise, transcranial magnetic stimulation, electroconvulsive therapy, brain imaging, genetic testing

Words and Phrases

1. Translate the following medical terms into Chinese or English.

1. 副作用   5. medical practice

2. 随机试验   6. selective serotonin reuptake inhibitors

3. 循证治疗   7. transcranial magnetic stimulation

4. 医学界   8. electroconvulsive therapy

II. Fill in the blanks with the words or phrases given below. Change the form if necessary.

1. conducive   4. accessibility

2. grapple   5. prescribed

3. alleviate

Sentence Translation

1. 该研究发现，在盲法试验中，心理疗法和抗抑郁药在减轻抑郁症状方面都比安慰剂更有效。然而，这两种治疗方法的疗效没有显著差异。

2. 心理疗法，如认知行为疗法（CBT）或心理动力学疗法（一种研究无意识情绪与痛苦症状之间相互作用的谈话疗法），可能会持续数月，包括长达数小时的疗程，这对许多人来说太过漫长。

3. 现代医疗实践中紧迫的时间和对行政管理的严格要求有时会导致患者预约匆忙，从而更偏向于提高效率和使用药物，而不是进行有意义的交谈讨论。

4. Cognitive behavioral therapy（CBT）teaches patients how to change negative patterns of thinking, feeling, and behaving that could exacerbate their depression.

5. The inclusion of additional examinations during doctors' visits may overlook the fundamental problem in the treatment of depression：do we allocate sufficient time to engage in meaningful conversations with our patients on their available choices?

Text B

After Reading Activities：

Reading Comprehension

Decide whether the following statements are true (T) or false (F) according to the text.

1. F   2. T   3. T   4. F   5. F

Match each English phrase in Column A with its Chinese version in Column B.

1. G   2. C   3. H   4. B   5. F   6. E   7. D   8. A

Translation

Commencing higher education represents a key transition point in a young person's life. It is a stage often accompanied by significant change combined with high expectations from students of what university life will be like, and also high expectations from themselves and others around on their academic performance. Relevant factors include moving away from home, learning to live independently, developing new social networks, adjusting to new ways of learning, and dealing with the additional and greater financial burdens. Higher education institutions have a unique opportunity to identify, prevent, and treat students' mental health problems because they provide support in multiple aspects of students' lives including academic studies, recreational activities, counselling services and residential accommodation.

Critical Thinking

When communicating with a friend who is experiencing severe anxiety due to the immense pressure at college, it is important to approach the conversation with empathy, understanding, and a non-judgmental attitude. Here are some suggestions for dealing with the anxiety and seeking appropriate help:

1. Listen actively: The first step in helping a friend who is struggling with anxiety is to listen actively. Let them know that you are there for them and that you care about their well-being. Encourage them to share their thoughts and feelings without interrupting or offering unsolicited advice.

2. Offer support: Let your friend know that you are willing to offer support in any way that you can. This could include accompanying them to therapy appointments, helping them find resources on campus, or simply being there to talk when they need someone to listen.

3. Encourage professional help: Anxiety can be a serious mental health condition that requires professional help. Encourage your friend to seek help from a therapist or counselor on campus or in the community. Offer to help them find a therapist or provide information about available resources.

4. Help them develop coping strategies: Encourage your friend to develop coping strategies that can help them manage their anxiety. This could include deep breathing exercises, meditation, yoga, or other relaxation techniques. You could also suggest that they engage in physical exercise or spend time doing activities that they enjoy.

5. Be patient: Remember that recovery from anxiety takes time and patience. Be patient with your friend as they work through their struggles and offer continued support and encouragement.

In conclusion, when communicating with a friend who is experiencing severe anxiety due to the immense pressure at college, it is important to listen actively, offer support, encourage professional help, help them develop coping strategies, and be patient. By doing so, you can help your friend manage their anxiety and seek the appropriate help they need to thrive.

Part III　Apply Medical English

Practical Activity

Doctor: Good morning, how can I assist you today?

Patient: Good morning. Recently, I've been experiencing some blurred vision and sensitivity to light. Can you help me with this?

Doctor: Sure, let's take a closer look. Have you experienced these symptoms before? And have you noticed any other changes in your vision?

Patient: No, this is the first time. Also, sometimes I feel a mild headache after prolonged reading or screen exposure.

Doctor: Based on your description, it could be a case of eye strain. But to be sure, we should conduct a thorough eye examination. This will help us identify the exact cause and suggest appropriate treatment.

Patient: That sounds reassuring. What tests will you perform?

Doctor: We'll start with a basic visual acuity test using an eye chart. Then, we'll check your eye pressure, examine the front part of your eye using a slit lamp, and dilate your pupils to inspect the retina and optic nerve at the back of the eye.

Patient: Alright, what if you find something abnormal?

Doctor: If we detect any abnormalities, such as signs of glaucoma, cataract, or age-related macular degeneration, we'll discuss the specific condition and potential treatment options. Depending on the disease, treatments might include medication, laser procedures, or surgery.

Patient: Thank you for explaining. When can I come in for the examination?

Doctor: Our next available appointment is in two days. Can you make it then? Also, please avoid wearing contact lenses for a week before the exam, as they can slightly alter the shape of your cornea and affect the accuracy of some tests.

Patient: Yes, that works for me. I'll refrain from wearing contacts as advised.

Doctor: Great! See you then. Remember, regular eye exams are essential for maintaining good eye health, even if you don't have any symptoms. It helps detect issues early on when they're most treatable.

Patient: I'll keep that in mind. Thank you for your time.

Doctor: You're welcome. Take care and see you soon.

B. Practical Unit Project

Script of a conversation between a doctor in psychiatry and a college student who has psychological problems:

Part I   Talking about Symptoms

Doctor: Hello! What seems to be the matter today?

Patient: Hello, doctor! I've been having these headaches just behind my eyes and I cannot sleep very well.

Doctor: How long have you been having them?

Patient: For about two weeks now. The headaches are not constant. They come and go but they are really painful. And I feel tired all the time for not getting enough sleep.

Doctor: Do you have a fever?

Patient: No, I don't think so.

Doctor: Is it the first time you are having these problems?

Patient: As far as I can remember, yes.

Doctor: OK, I need to check your pulse and blood pressure. I'll also need to check your lymph nodes to see if they are swollen.

(a few minutes later)

Doctor: Well, I don't see anything physically wrong with you. May I ask what prevents you from sleeping well? Is there anything bothering you?

Patient: Well, I am a freshman and I can't adapt to my new college life quite well. There are so many things to worry about. For example, there are many different lectures I have to attend. I need to do my laundry by myself, the food in our canteen is not as tasty as my mom's home cooking. Besides, I don't get along with my roommates very well.

Part II   Giving Advice and Prescribing Medicine

Doctor: I understand that college life can be very challenging for freshmen, and you've been experiencing a lot of changes.

Patient: What should I do, doctor?

Doctor: Well, I suggest that you call your old friends or talk to them online. Also, don't just stay in your dorm. Try joining some clubs or attending activities you like. In your spare time, you'd better do some mild exercise like jogging or swimming. Don't just focus on your grades but pay more attention to the learning process instead. Are you currently taking any medication?

Patient: No, I am not taking any.

Doctor: Any allergies?

Patient: No.

Doctor: I'm going to prescribe you some painkillers. Take them as soon as you feel your headaches are starting. If you are still in pain after an hour, take the second one. Don't take more than 2 pills in 4 hours, or more than 6 pills in a 24-hour period.

Patient: OK.

Doctor: Please don't drink any alcohol while you are taking these pills, or they might not be that effective.

Patient: Could I get my body checked? What if it gets more serious?

Doctor: If you still have the same problem in two weeks, then we will need to investigate further. I am sure it will be all cleared up soon.

Patient: Do I have to pay for the prescription?

Doctor: You should pay a 10-pound prescription fee. These pills will be enough for a month.

Patient: Can I take this prescription to any chemist's?

Doctor: Yes, of course. There's a chemist shop near the supermarket around the corner. You can get your medicine there.

Patient: OK, I'll do that. Thank you!

Doctor: No problem. I wish you to recover as soon as possible!

Unit 6   Keys to Exercises and Audio Scripts

Part I   View the Medical World

1. A   2. A   3. C   4. C   5. D

Script

When was the last time you had a difficult interaction with an angry or upset patient? You felt ambushed, didn't know what to do or say. It did not go well and you felt bad for days... This is Doctor Dike Drummond at *thehappyMD.com* and in this short video, I'm going to show you a way to deal with angry and upset patients quickly, efficiently, effectively, empathetically and get on with your office day in home on time. I call it the Universal Upset Person Protocol. See most of us don't get any training on how to deal with emotionally upset or angry patients, so we do what comes naturally. We either try to fix their problem or we try to defend ourselves or whatever the upset person is upset about and that's just about as effective as throwing gas on a fire. Here's why. See in an ordinary office visit where the patient's not upset, you can talk about what brought them in, but if they're upset, there's a lot of emotion in the room. It's feelings first. They simply have to share their feelings and feel understood and listened to before they can go any farther. Teddy Roosevelt once said, "People don't care how much you know until they know how much you care." It's exactly like that. And the Universal Upset Person Protocol is the quickest way to give the patient a safe place to vent their feelings, share them with you. You'd listen so you can wrap it up and move into the clinical part of your office visit. Let me take you through the six steps of the protocol real quickly here in an overview and then we'll go into them in more depth in just a minute. And just so you know, down below the video frame here is a handout that gives you a full training including all the statements and questions in the protocol. Make sure you get that before you're done here today. Here are the six steps:

Number one: You look really upset.

Number two: Tell me about it.

Number three: I'm so sorry that this is happening to you.

Number four: What would you like me to do to help you.

Number five: Here's what I'd like us to do next.

Number six: Thank you so much for sharing your feelings with me. It's really important that we understand each other completely. Thank you.

Now let's drop down and go through those one at a time. Upset patients come in two flavors usually. One they're obvious and they're verbal, you can hear them coming down the hallway; second type are quiet and see things. They don't speak but everybody knows they're upset. Either way, if you notice this, you're not going anywhere till they clear these emotions, so your first statement is "You look really upset". You'll typically get one of two responses: "You bet, I am." is one and the second one is "I'm not upset, I'm frustrated." Or they may name some other emotion like that. Now there's a piece inside of you that may feel bad. You may feel like you got it wrong. You can let that go. Your observation has caused them to look inside and get clear on what they're really feeling. That's the first thing they have to do. So great job.

Here's step number two: Tell me about it. What you've done is going to give them a green light to tell you their experience. And your job is to listen. You are to understand what they're going through and make sure they notice that you're listening. They feel heard.

And here's step number three: no matter what's happened, you can apologize: I'm so sorry that you're feeling this way. I'm so sorry this is happening to you. Let them know that you have sympathy for their situation. Critically important to maintaining your bond with this patient.

There's the next step: What would you like me to do to help you. And here again you've got to listen and as you're listening this time, notice your boundaries. Notice things that the patient may request that you're not comfortable with.

Next step. When they're done, take a pause. Think about what you're willing to do and tell them here's what I'm willing to do for going forward. Here's what I suggest. Here's a plan I recommend and any time that you are not giving them something they've requested, tell them what you are going to do instead.

And last, to wrap this difficult encounter up in a way that builds your relationship for the long term, thank them for being willing to share their feelings with you. Let them know how important it is that you understand each other clearly.

There you go six steps to the Universal Upset Person Protocol and this works with anybody who's upset: your children, your significant other, your colleagues, your staff, random people on the street will respond to you much more positively and go breezing right through their upset when you use the protocol.

Part II   Read to Explore Medical Knowledge

Text A

After Reading Activities:

Reading Comprehension

I. Answer the following questions.

1. The significance of clear, concise, and empathetic communication between patients and their health care providers was brought to my attention when I received an unexpected breast cancer diagnosis.

2. It could change the perception of a potentially fatal diagnosis into an unexpectedly beneficial educational opportunity, thereby easing the burden brought by the diagnosis and the treatment's adverse effects, and making the patient's adherence to therapy easier.

3. Poor communication may lead to medication errors, which frequently result in negative outcomes or even death. Besides, patients may sue for medical malpractice because of misunderstanding on the part of doctors caused by poor communication. Furthermore, it may have devastating effects on the doctor's practice and reputation.

4. Skills such as: Exhibit patience and attentiveness towards both the spoken and unspoken aspects of the patient's communication. Show interest in talking to patients through mannerisms, body language, and active involvement, such as leaning towards them. Listen carefully and be sure not to interrupt when the patient is telling something. Always offer helpful information when necessary and quickly respond to the patient's reaction. Articles, brochures, and FAQs should be provided in case serious and chronic diseases are diagnosed. Discuss the disease's nature, course, prognosis, treatment options, and the need for investigations, etc. Discuss the necessity and feasibility of expensive investigations and drugs and their effect on main course and outcome of disease. Get the patient involved in the decision-making. The treatment plan must conform to the patient's cognition. Make extra efforts into encouraging patients regarding adherence to lifestyle changes. Use simple language instead of medical jargon.

5. The COVID-19 epidemic has brought about a shift in the conventional face-to-face patient-physician contact. Since patients and physicians are physically separated, telemedicine technology needed to advance quickly to provide consultations. This raised a number of ethical concerns but also presented a myriad of potential to enhance and broaden communication channels.

II. Work in groups to complete the following chart according to the structure of the text.

Concerns over doctor-patient relationship: (paras. 1-2)

Publications,

My experience of encountering with health care professionals (paras. 3-6)

because of my unpleasant experiences with health care professionals, the importance of effective communication,

My thoughts about doctor-patient communication during the process of treating breast cancer (paras. 7-19)

a trustworthy and meaningful relationship, the COVID-19 pandemic, virtual communication,

Conclusion: (para. 20)

the conventional principles

Words and Phrases

I. Translate the following medical terms into Chinese or English.

1. 有效的医患沟通
2. 建立可信且有意义的关系
3. 临床效果不佳
4. 患者不切实际的期望

5. enhance and broaden communication channels
6. health care provider's mumblings
7. diagnosis and treatment plan
8. feasibility of investigations

II. Fill in the blanks with the words or phrases given below. Change the form if necessary.

1. perceptions
2. mitigate
3. unfaltering

4. empathetic
5. consultation

Sentence Translation

1. 该技术优化并支持整个患者护理过程，并实现了医疗系统内医患之间信息交流的畅通，从而更容易启动、监控和记录医患之间的交流。

2. 由于患者和医生之间存在物理距离，远程医疗技术需要迅速发展以提供咨询服务。这引发了许多伦理问题，但也呈现了增强和拓宽沟通渠道的多种可能性。

3. 研究表明非语言沟通确实会影响患者满意度，但人们普遍认为其重要性不如语言沟通。

4. Discuss the necessity and feasibility of expensive investigations and drugs and their effect on main course and outcome of disease.

5. Health care professionals must adjust and acquire the skills to minimize the potential hazards of digital communication with their patients.

Text B

After Reading Activities：

Reading Comprehension

Decide whether the following statements are true (T) or false (F) according to the text.

1. T   2. T   3. F   4. F   5. T

Match each English phrase in Column A with its Chinese version in Column B.

1. H   2. B   3. A   4. G   5. C   6. F   7. E   8. D

Translation

I have been working for 9 years to promote bedside exam skills, which emphasizes the importance of personal interactions for both diagnostics and for building trust between the physician and patient. When a trainee seeks my advice about a patient, my first answer is, "We can't make that decision now. We need to see the patient first." You can learn so much stuff that's between the lines. How much distress are they really in? Can they really not breathe? Can they talk to me in full sentences? How weak are they? I'm really trying to get a sense of the person. That's when the decision-making just gets a lot better.

Critical Thinking

Possible answer: Yes, it is true that burnout is a significant factor preventing doctors from spending adequate time listening to their patients. Burnout among physicians is a well-documented issue, characterized by emotional exhaustion, depersonalization, and a reduced sense of personal accomplishment. This state of chronic stress can lead to decreased quality of care, reduced patient satisfaction, and higher rates of medical errors.

To help address the problem of physician burnout and improve doctor-patient communication, several strategies can be implemented：

1. Improving Work Environment

2. Promoting Work-Life Balance

3. Providing Mental Health Support

4. Fostering a Supportive Culture

5. Investing in Technology

6. Training and Education

7. Patient-Centered Care Models

By implementing these strategies, health care systems can help reduce physician burnout, allowing doctors to spend more meaningful time with their patients and improving overall health care outcomes.

Part III   Apply Medical English

Practical Activity

Doctor-Patient Dialogue: Stomatology

Scene: Dental Clinic

Dr. Lee (Dentist): Good afternoon, Mr. Anderson. What brings you in today?

Mr. Anderson (Patient): Good afternoon, Dr. Lee. I've been having a lot of pain in my mouth, especially when I eat or drink something hot or cold. It's been really bothering me for the past week.

Dr. Lee: I'm sorry to hear that. Let's take a closer look. Can you tell me if the pain is localized to a specific area or if it's more general?

Mr. Anderson: The pain is mostly around my back teeth, on the left side. It feels like it's coming from one of my molars.

Dr. Lee: I see. Have you noticed any swelling, bleeding gums, or bad breath?

Mr. Anderson: Yes, my gums have been bleeding a bit when I brush, and my breath doesn't seem fresh, even right after brushing.

Dr. Lee: Thank you for sharing that. Let me examine your mouth. Please open wide.

[*Dr. Lee examines Mr. Anderson's mouth with a dental mirror and probe.*]

Dr. Lee: It looks like you have a cavity in one of your molars, and your gums are quite inflamed. This could be causing your pain and bleeding. The cavity might have reached the pulp of the tooth, which is why you're experiencing sensitivity to hot and cold.

Mr. Anderson: That sounds serious. What can we do about it?

Dr. Lee: The first step is to treat the cavity. Given the severity, you might need a root canal to remove the infected pulp and save the tooth. After that, we'll fill the cavity and possibly place a crown to protect the tooth. As for your gums, it looks like you have gingivitis, which is the inflammation of the gums.

Mr. Anderson: A root canal? I've heard those can be painful.

Dr. Lee: It's a common concern, but modern techniques have made root canals much more comfortable than they used to be. We'll make sure you're properly anesthetized, and you shouldn't feel any pain during the procedure. Post-procedure discomfort can usually be managed with over-the-counter pain relievers.

Mr. Anderson: Okay, that's reassuring. And what about my gums?

Dr. Lee: For your gums, a professional cleaning will help remove plaque and tartar buildup. I'll also give you some tips on maintaining good oral hygiene to prevent gingivitis from returning. Regular brushing, flossing, and using an antiseptic mouthwash can make a big difference.

Mr. Anderson: Thank you, Dr. Lee. How soon can we start the treatments?

Dr. Lee: We can schedule the root canal for later this week, and I recommend starting with a deep cleaning today to address the gingivitis. After the root canal, we'll place the filling and crown in subsequent visits. Does that work for you?

Mr. Anderson: Yes, that works for me. I'm eager to get this pain sorted out.

Dr. Lee: Great. We'll take good care of you. Let's begin with the cleaning today, and I'll have my assistant help you schedule the root canal.

Mr. Anderson: Thank you, Dr. Lee. I appreciate your help.

Dr. Lee: You're welcome, Mr. Anderson. Let's get started on your cleaning now, and we'll get you back to feeling comfortable and healthy.

[*Dr. Lee begins the cleaning procedure, explaining each step to Mr. Anderson to keep him informed and comfortable.*]

B. Practical Unit Project

Essay:

Effective communication between doctors and patients is crucial for delivering high-quality health care. Clear, empathetic interaction not only enhances patient satisfaction but also improves treatment adherence and health outcomes. Here are several practical strategies for fostering better doctor-patient communication.

Firstly, Doctors should practice active listening, which involves giving full attention to the patient, avoiding interruptions, and responding thoughtfully. This ensures that patients feel heard and understood, fostering trust and openness.

Secondly, showing empathy is a good method, which involves recognizing and validating patients' feelings and concerns. A compassionate approach can make patients feel more comfortable discussing sensitive issues, which is essential for accurate diagnosis and effective treatment.

Finally, non-verbal communication such as body language, eye contact, and facial expressions play a significant role in communication. Positive non-verbal cues can convey attentiveness and concern, while negative cues can create barriers.

By integrating these strategies, health care providers can create a more effective and compassionate communication environment, ultimately leading to better patient care and outcomes.

Unit 7　Keys to Exercises and Audio Scripts

Part I　View the Medical World

1. C　2. B　3. A　4. D　5. A

Script

You've probably heard this conversation starter many times before: "Tell me about yourself." You might answer with your name, where you're from, and maybe a fun fact. Whether you've thought about these details deeply or not, they lay the foundation of a story that reflects you. The building of this story plays a critical role in narrative medicine. Narrative medicine is the practice of mindfully contextualizing a patient's lived experiences to better care for and treat them. It's an approach to health care that considers not only the physical, but also the mental and emotional aspects of a person's health. By seeking out a patient's story, clinicians can gain an in-depth perspective of their patient, and ultimately see a whole person, not just a diagnosis. Narrative medicine requires a vast array of skills—clinicians must be able to listen to, comprehend, and act upon a patient's story. Sometimes, a patient's story isn't clean-cut, so clinicians also need to be able to navigate its nuances. This set of skills is called narrative competence, and clinicians can improve their narrative competence through creative expression. Narrative medicine provides a solution to common challenges faced by clinicians and patients. A clinician cannot rely on their medical knowledge alone to prevent, diagnose, and treat illnesses. If they cannot communicate and connect with their patient, the patient may feel neglected, invalidated, or even hesitant to return for another visit. In some cases, a clinician may miss the correct diagnosis, or the prescribed treatment may be ineffective. If a patient is from a marginalized population that has suffered historical, racial or other categorical trauma, the disconnect can be even larger. The most common sources of disconnect between a clinician and a patient are known as the "four divides". These are obstacles that hamper the development of a strong, patient-clinician connection. The first divide is differing views on mortality. While clinicians primarily encounter illness and death through their work, patients often react more strongly based on their personal experiences. The second divide is the context of illness. Most clinicians see illness as a phenomenon requiring medical intervention, while a patient may see illness as the effect it has on their life and on others. The third divide is differing beliefs about the causes of disease. Not only do clinicians have extensive medical training, but their knowledge is also valued more than their patient's, creating an unequal balance. The final divide is vulnerability. Patients may be hesitant to share personal details about their lives, and a clinician may be hesitant to inquire, making the process of diagnosis and treatment more difficult and stressful. Through conversations, narrative medicine can result in more personalized care with improved health outcomes.

Part II　Read to Explore Medical Knowledge

Text A

After Reading Activities:

Reading Comprehension

I. Answer the following questions.

1. Present century is probably the best time to respond prudently. For one thing, the greatest scientific discoveries in every discipline have been achieved in the last hundred years, yet modernism has also altered the nature of time. The creation of goods and information, the dissemination of information, the development of interpersonal relationships, and the rate of communication unfold at rates that were previously inconceivable. For another thing, it is

undeniable that the 20th century was a watershed moment in medical history.

2. Fordist Logic means "Produce more and more in less time" appears to be the mantra. Being "better" requires us to be productive. There are a number of areas that have been significantly expedited, including the development of new diagnostic tests, surgeries, and medications, as well as the rapid response to medical emergencies. However, it appears that all aspects of life, including what must inevitably be put on hold, are being swept along by these benefits.

3. First, a medical practice that is imbued with storytelling abilities that enable doctors to hear, understand, and be moved by patients' stories—all while maintaining a framework of respect for the individual impacted by the illness—and second, the cultivation of medical professionals through the experiences gained from this approach to the patient.

4. One the one hand, the incommunicable may be partially due to the personality of the patients who are usually shy and introverted, reluctant to communicate with strangers. On the other hand, it may have something to do with the disease, be it a family heredity or something unpleasant concerning the experience of contracting the diseases or the social stigma that may endanger their daily life.

5. The doctor-patient relationship has been strengthened, clinical analysis of the cases studied has improved, and our understanding of disease diagnosis, prognosis, and therapy has deepened as a result of this technique. Furthermore, it can enhance the patient's involvement in shared decision-making processes.

II. Work in groups to complete the following chart according to the structure of the text.

Modernity is a double-edged sword. (paras. 1-2)

scientific breakthroughs, the Renaissance, the modern day, a watershed moment, the creation of goods and information, the development of interpersonal relationships, the rate of communication, the relationship between doctors and their patients

Problems occur when doctors ignore patients' experience and internal world. (paras. 3-5)

statistics, income, patient's experience and inner world, doctor-patient interaction, healing skills, a loving attitude, imbued with storytelling abilities, the cultivation of medical professionals

What can doctors do to cope with the problem? (paras. 6-8)

pedestal, language that both parties can understand, impersonal objects

Conclusion: the advantages of using the narrative techniques in the field of medical education (para. 9)

using the narrative medicine

Words and Phrases

I. Translate the following medical terms into Chinese or English.

1. 叙事医学   5. rapid response to medical emergencies

2. 医患关系   6. diagnosis and treatment of illness

3. 改进临床分析   7. the cultivation of medical professionals

4. 道德准则   8. medical intervention

II. Fill in the blanks with the words or phrases given below. Change the form if necessary.

1. unfolded   4. prudent

2. insistence on   5. medications

3. antagonistic

Sentence Translation

1. 医生无法进入无法沟通或极难沟通的领域，除非他们成为患者的旅伴，陪伴他们进行探索，并找到一种生动、准确和具有隐喻性的语言来描述那些似乎无法沟通的东西。

2. 这种叙事实践包括两个步骤：首先，一种充满讲故事能力的医疗实践，使医生能够听懂、理解病人的故事并被病人的故事所感动——同时尊重受疾病影响的个体；其次，用这种治疗患者的方法所获得的经验，来培养医疗专业人员。

3. 商品和信息的创造，人际关系的发展以及沟通的速度都以以前难以想象的速度展开。

4. Narrative medicine was established to return to a fuller picture of the patient. Dr. Rita Charon came up with this word, and it's meant to provide an alternative perspective to present orthodoxy.

5. The service time is becoming shorter due to the necessity of attending to a specific number of patients per hour. The patient is not thoroughly evaluated, and in exchange, a battery of imaging and laboratory testing is sought in order to arrive at a diagnosis.

Text B

After Reading Activities:

Reading Comprehension

Decide whether the following statements are true (T) or false (F) according to the text.

1. T　2. F　3. F　4. F　5. T

Match each English phrase in Column A with its Chinese version in Column B.

1. D　2. C　3. A　4. G　5. H　6. F　7. E　8. B

Translation

　　Narrative medicine is a medical practice and educational approach that aims to improve medical personnel's ability to care for patients, empathize with them, and think medically by drawing on literary and narrative techniques. It emphasizes that health care professionals should not only focus on patients' physical symptoms and medical history, but also understand their personal stories, backgrounds and emotional experiences to gain a more complete understanding of patients' needs and concerns. Narrative medicine texts bridge the gap between medical terminology and human emotion, allowing patients to share their experiences and health care professionals to listen and understand.

Critical Thinking

　　To conduct a study assessing the impact of narrative medicine techniques on enhancing communication between health care providers and patients, we can follow a qualitative research approach utilizing interviews and surveys to gather patients' perceptions. Here's a proposed study design:

　　Study Design:

　　Objective:

　　To assess the impact of incorporating narrative medicine techniques on enhancing communication between health care providers and patients.

　　Methodology:

　　Participant Selection:

　　Select a diverse sample of patients from various health care settings (e.g., hospitals, clinics) who have experienced narrative medicine techniques during their interactions with health care providers.

Ensure representation across different demographic factors such as age, gender, ethnicity, and medical conditions.

Data Collection:

Conduct semi-structured interviews with selected patients to explore their experiences and perceptions of interactions with health care providers using narrative medicine techniques. Questions can focus on the effectiveness of narrative medicine in fostering empathy, understanding, and trust, as well as any perceived improvements in communication and patient-provider relationships.

Administer surveys to a larger sample of patients who have encountered narrative medicine techniques to gather quantitative data on their overall satisfaction and perceived impact on communication. Include Likert scale questions and open-ended items to capture nuanced responses.

By conducting this study, we aim to contribute valuable insights into the role of narrative medicine in fostering meaningful connections between health care providers and patients, ultimately enhancing the quality of patient care and satisfaction.

Part III   Apply Medical English

Practical Activity

Doctor (Dr. Patel): Good morning, Mrs. Johnson. What brings you in today?

Patient (Mrs. Johnson): Good morning, Dr. Patel. I've been having some issues with my ears lately.

Dr. Patel: I see. Can you tell me more about what you've been experiencing?

Mrs. Johnson: Well, I've been having a lot of pain in my left ear, and it feels like it's blocked. I've also been having some trouble hearing.

Dr. Patel: I'm sorry to hear that. Let's take a look and see what's going on. (*Dr. Patel examines Mrs. Johnson's ears.*) Ah, I see some inflammation and fluid buildup in your left ear. It looks like you have an ear infection.

Mrs. Johnson: Oh no, how did that happen?

Dr. Patel: Ear infections can occur for various reasons, such as bacterial or viral infections, allergies, or even trapped water in the ear canal. But the good news is, we can treat it.

Mrs. Johnson: What do we need to do?

Dr. Patel: I'll prescribe some antibiotics to help clear up the infection. You may also benefit from using some ear drops to help reduce the inflammation and relieve the pain.

Mrs. Johnson: Will I need to come back for a follow-up?

Dr. Patel: Yes, I'd like to see you back in about a week to make sure the infection is clearing up and to check your hearing. If you experience any worsening symptoms or if the pain doesn't improve, please give us a call.

Mrs. Johnson: Okay, thank you, Dr. Patel.

Dr. Patel: Before you go, do you have any other concerns or symptoms you'd like to discuss?

Mrs. Johnson: Actually, I've also been experiencing some nasal congestion and post-nasal drip lately.

Dr. Patel: That's important information. Nasal congestion and post-nasal drip can sometimes be related to ear infections, especially if they're caused by allergies or sinus issues. Let's discuss that further after we address your ear infection.

Mrs. Johnson: Sounds good. Thank you for your help, Dr. Patel.

Dr. Patel: You're welcome, Mrs. Johnson. Let's get you started on the treatment plan, and we'll take it from there.

B. Practical Unit Project

Dear [Classmate's Name],

I hope this letter finds you well. As we continue our journey through medical school, I wanted to share a memorable doctor-patient story from my recent internship experience that left a lasting impact on me.

During my time in the hospital, I had the privilege of assisting Dr. Alvarez, an experienced oncologist, in caring for a patient named Mr. Thompson. Mr. Thompson was a middle-aged man diagnosed with advanced-stage lung cancer. Despite his grim prognosis, he maintained a positive attitude and showed remarkable resilience throughout his treatment journey.

What struck me most about Mr. Thompson was his unwavering determination to fight his illness while maintaining a sense of dignity and grace. Despite the physical and emotional toll of his cancer treatment, he always greeted us with a smile and expressed gratitude for the care he received.

One particular moment stands out vividly in my memory. During one of his chemotherapy sessions, Mr. Thompson took the time to ask Dr. Alvarez about her own well-being and thanked her for her dedication to his care. Despite facing his own mortality, he remained empathetic and compassionate towards others, including the medical staff.

Mr. Thompson's story taught me valuable lessons about the resilience of the human spirit and the importance of compassionate care in medicine. His positive outlook and unwavering spirit continue to inspire me as I navigate my own journey in health care.

I wanted to share this story with you as a reminder of the profound impact we can have on our patients' lives, even in the face of adversity. I look forward to hearing about your own experiences and insights as we continue our medical education together.

Warm regards,

[Your Name]

Unit 8　Keys to Exercises and Audio Scripts

Part I　View the Medical World

1. D　2. A　3. B　4. A　5. C

Script

"Hello! I'm Pepper. Can I help you with something?"

It is easy to see why this humanoid robot got the job as the newest staff member at Belgium's AZ Damiaan hospital. Pepper speaks nineteen languages, knows her way around the place, and has the perfect bedside manner. Employed to welcome patients and visitors, it was developed by Belgium's Zora Bots to improve health care. The company's Fabrice Goffin says Pepper is unlike other humanoid robots on the market.

"The robot itself is a meter and twenty high, so it is not like Arnold Schwarzenegger with a leather jacket and an 'I will be back' robot. It is a quite nice robot and the reactions are positive for the moment for as long as it doesn't take jobs, but it is not the case for Pepper."

The robot was designed with specialized software that works on any device with Internet access. A complete charge gives it up to twenty hours of walk and talk time, and at a mellow pace of three kilometers per hour, all patients are able to keep up with Pepper, even slower moving ones.

In its first week on the job, Pepper was assigned to the maternity ward.

"It is another way of making contact and maybe it is reassuring that it is a robot for some people. So it can be, I know. The baby was reassured; he didn't mind (I'm sorry) putting his hands on it. It didn't frighten him, so I think it will be important, especially for children."

With a personal touch like Pepper's, heading to the hospital could become a new kind of experience, one that even puts a smile on patients' faces.

Part II Read to Explore Medical Knowledge

Text A

After Reading Activities:

Reading Comprehension

I. Answer the following questions.

1. AI system can optimize the doctors' schedule by guiding the doctor to the most logical assignment so as to help both patients and doctors reduce waiting time.

2. A million pages can be processed in seconds by IBM Watson. Due to its impressive speed, Watson is now being tested at oncology centers to assess its usefulness in cancer treatment decision-making.

3. IBM Watson enables professionals to access evidence-based treatment alternatives. Advanced data analysis capabilities in Watson for Oncology allow it to make sense of clinical notes and reports containing both structured and unstructured data, which could be essential when choosing a treatment course.

4. AI can help doctors do administrative work. It can learn how to do it properly and do it better than doctors by time.

5. Instead of replacing doctors, AI will augment them and make them better at their jobs. By eliminating the day-to-day treadmill of administrative and repetitive duties, the medical community would be able to fully dedicate their attention to their primary objective: healing.

II. Work in groups to complete the following chart according to the structure of the text.

Introduction: (para. 1)

health care systems, the "average doctor"

Body part: (paras. 2-16)

patients, medical professionals, in line with, pinpoint accuracy, AI operating system, pertinent, device, diagnosis, notice, challenging, extending invitations to collaborate, administrative

Conclusion：(para. 17)

augment，healing

Words and Phrases

I. Translate the following medical terms into Chinese or English.

1. 医疗专业人员

2. 认知助手

3. 医学界

4. 治疗这种疾病

5. AI operating system

6. oncology center

7. clinical report

8. treatment course

II. Fill in the blanks with the words or phrases given below. Change the form if necessary.

1. Suboptimal

2. clinical

3. monotonous

4. privilege

5. condition

Sentence Translation

1. 不理想的医疗流程既导致病人在医生办公室前长时间等候，也导致医务人员每天由于例如等待病人或检查结果等各种因素浪费大量时间。

2. 通过识别医生、诊所或医院在治疗相同病症时是否会犯同样的错误，它们可以帮助医疗机构改善患者护理，减少可避免的住院治疗。

3. 该项目旨在构建一个复杂的"认知助手"，它拥有先进的分析和推理能力，以及丰富的治疗知识。

4. Think about how much easier and more effective it would be if digital communication were in line with our specific needs，allowing us to send and receive information with pinpoint accuracy and no effort.

5. Advanced data analysis capabilities allow it to make sense of clinical notes and reports containing both structured and unstructured data，which could be essential when choosing a treatment course.

Text B

After Reading Activities：

Reading Comprehension

Decide whether the following statements are true (T) or false (F) according to the text.

1. T   2. T   3. F   4. F   5. F

Match each English phrase in Column A with its Chinese version in Column B.

1. H   2. F   3. E   4. B   5. D   6. A   7. C   8. G

Translation

Today, as we enter the stage of artificial intelligence development, people often ask, will artificial intelligence replace doctors when technology is so advanced and can solve so many problems? Artificial intelligence can improve health care, but it cannot replace doctors. According to our definition of health care, health care is not just equal to medical technology services; health care is medical technology plus medical humanities. Because medicine is not only a science, but also a sociology, the sentiment of medical humanities is timeless. We need to integrate medical humanities into the development of technology, especially artificial intelligence, to make these high-tech products more humane.

Critical Thinking

With the advancement of AI in medical field, it is true that there might be a psychological gap between doctors and patients. However, there are several ways to bridge this gap while still utilizing the benefits of AI in health care.

1. Human touch: Even with AI's involvement, it is important for doctors to maintain a human touch in their interactions with patients. This can be achieved by being empathetic, listening actively, and providing emotional support to patients.

2. Personalized care: AI can help doctors provide personalized care by analyzing patient data and recommending tailored treatment plans. This will make patients feel more valued and understood, thereby reducing the psychological gap.

3. Clear communication: Doctors should clearly communicate the role of AI in the diagnosis and treatment process to patients. This will help patients understand the importance of AI and how it complements the doctor's expertise, rather than replacing it.

4. Training and education: Doctors can bridge the gap by educating themselves on the latest AI technologies and their applications in health care. This will enable them to better explain the benefits and limitations of AI to their patients.

5. Collaborative decision-making: Involving patients in the decision-making process can help bridge the psychological gap. By using AI to analyze patient data and presenting the results to the patient, doctors can involve patients in the decision-making process, making them feel more involved and valued.

6. Continuous monitoring: AI can help doctors monitor patients' health continuously, allowing

for early detection of any issues. This will help patients feel more secure and confident in their doctor's ability to provide timely and effective care.

7. Patient feedback: Encouraging patients to provide feedback on their experience with AI-assisted health care can help doctors identify areas of improvement and address any concerns or misconceptions patients may have.

In conclusion, while AI has its advantages in the medical field, it is essential for doctors to maintain a strong connection with their patients. By incorporating the above strategies, we can bridge the psychological gap and provide high-quality, patient-centered care.

Part III   Apply Medical English

Practical Activity

Doctor: Hi, how can I help you today?

Patient: Hi, I'm not feeling well. I have a really bad headache and my stomach is upset.

Doctor: I'm sorry to hear that. Have you been experiencing these symptoms for a while or did they just come on suddenly?

Patient: They just came on suddenly. I was fine this morning, but then my head started hurting and my stomach felt queasy.

Doctor: I see. Have you been under any stress lately or had any recent changes in your diet or routine?

Patient: Not really. Everything has been pretty normal.

Doctor: Alright. Based on your symptoms, it's possible that you may be experiencing a migraine or a gastrointestinal issue. I'll need to do some tests to determine the exact cause. In the meantime, I can give you something to help with the pain and discomfort.

Patient: Thank you, doctor. That would be really helpful.

Doctor: You're welcome. Before we proceed, do you have any other symptoms or medical conditions that I should be aware of?

Patient: No, I don't think so. I'm generally healthy and don't take any medications.

Doctor: Okay, good to know. Please follow me to the examination room, and we'll get started with the tests. In the meantime, try to rest and drink plenty of fluids.

Patient: Alright, thank you, doctor.

Doctor: You're welcome. We'll do our best to get you feeling better soon.

B. Practical Unit Project（略）

Glossary

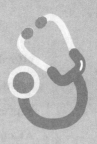

affordability *n.* 可购性;负担能力	3 Part II A
agent *n.* 药剂;药物	1 Part II A
aggregate *v.* 总计	1 Part II A
AI operating system 人工智能操作系统	8 Part II A
AI-backed *adj.* 人工智能技术支持的	8 Part II B
ailment *n.* 疾病;小病	4 Part II B
aim *v.* 力求达到;力争做到	8 Part II A
algae *n.* 海藻	2 Part II B
alginate *n.* 海藻盐酸	2 Part II B
algorithm *n.* 算法;计算程序	8 Part II B
allergist *n.* 过敏症专科医生	7 Part III
allergy *n.* 过敏	4 Part I
alleviate *v.* 减轻;缓和;缓解	4 Part III
alternative *n.* 可供选择的事物	2 Part II B
alternative therapy 替代疗法	4 Part II B
ambushed *adj.* 中埋伏的	6 Part I
amendable *adj.* 改善的	3 Part II A
ample *adj.* 足够的;丰裕的	1 Part II B
an array of 一系列;大量的	7 Part I
anatomy *n.* 解剖学	7 Part II B
antagonistic *adj.* 敌对的;敌意的	7 Part II A
antibiotics *n.* 抗菌素;抗生素	1 Part II B
antidepressant *n.* 抗抑郁药	5 Part II A
anti-histamines *n.* 抗组胺剂	4 Part II A
anti-inflammatory *adj.* 抗炎的;消炎的	2 Part II A
antiviral *adj.* 抗病毒的	3 Part II B
apolipoprotein *n.* 载脂蛋白	2 Part II A
appendicitis *n.* 阑尾炎	4 Part II B
appreciate *v.* 感激	6 Part III
approach *n.* 方法;途径	7 Part II B
appropriate *v.* 盗用;挪用;占用;侵吞	7 Part II A

approximately *adv.* 大概;大约   3 Part II B

arising *adj.* 发生的;出现的   8 Part II A

arrhythmia *n.* 心律失常;心律不齐   1 Part II A

arthritis *n.* [外科]关节炎   3 Part I

artificial intelligence   人工智能   8 Part II A

as opposed to   而不是   5 Part II A

aspirin *n.* 阿司匹林(镇痛解热消炎药)   8 Part II B

assess *v.* 评估;评定(性质、质量)   8 Part II B

assign *v.* 指定;指派   8 Part I

associate *adj.* (常用于头衔)非正式的;准的;副的   1 Part II B

asymptomatic *adj.* 无临床症状的   1 Part II A

augment *v.* 增加;提高;扩大   8 Part II A

auscultation *n.* 听诊   4 Part II B

autonomy *n.* 自主;自主权   6 Part II B

awe-inspiring *adj.* 令人惊叹的;使人敬佩的;令人敬慕的   5 Part II B

baffle *v.* 使困惑;难住   3 Part II A

ballgame *n.* 情况;局面   6 Part II B

bipartisan *adj.* 两党的;涉及两党的   3 Part II A

blinded trial *n.* 盲法试验   5 Part II A

blood clot *n.* 血栓   4 Part II A

blood pressure cuff[医]血压表套袖   8 Part II B

blood vessel *n.* 血管   5 Part II B

bolster *v.* 改善;加强   1 Part II B

breastfeed infant   母乳喂养的婴儿   2 Part III

breeze through 轻松地做某事   6 Part I

brochure *n.* 资料(或广告)手册   6 Part II A

burnout *n.* 精疲力竭;过度劳累   3 Part II A

byzantine *adj.* 拜占庭帝国的;东罗马帝国的;(思想、制度等)复杂神秘
而死板的   3 Part II A

calibrate *v.* 精确测量;准确估量   1 Part II A

caloric *adj.* 热量的   2 Part II A

cap *v.* 限额收取（或支出）	3 Part II B
capitaliz *v.* 变现	5 Part II B
capsule *n.* 胶囊	4 Part II B
cardiac *adj.* 心脏的；心脏病的	5 Part II B
cardiometabolic *adj.* 心血管代谢的	2 Part II A
cardioscope *n.* 心脏示波器；心脏镜；心电图示波器	7 Part II A
cardiovascular *adj.* 心血管的	2 Part II A
catalog *n.* 目录；目录簿	3 Part II B
catch-all term 万能术语	4 Part II B
categorical trauma 范畴性创伤	7 Part I
cavity *n.* 蛀牙	6 Part III
cerebrospinal *adj.* 脑脊液的	2 Part I
charge *n.* 充电量	8 Part I
chemotherapy *n.* （尤指对癌的）化学治疗；化学疗法；化疗	6 Part II B
cholesterol *n.* 胆固醇	4 Part II A
chronic *adj.* 长期的；慢性的；难以治愈（或根除）的	1 Part II A
chronic pain 慢性疼痛	4 Part I
chronic ailment 慢性疾病	1 Part III
chronological *adj.* 按时间计算的（年龄）（相对于身体、智力或情感等方面的发展而言）	2 Part II A
circulate *v.* 传播	1 Part II A
claim *v.* 索要；索取	3 Part III
clinician *n.* 临床医师	6 Part II B
cluster *n.* 团；群；簇	1 Part II A
coexisting *adj.* 共存的	1 Part II A
cognition *n.* 认知	2 Part II A
cognitive *adj.* 认知的；感知的；认识的	5 Part II A
cohort *n.* （有共同特点或举止类同的）一群人	2 Part II A
collaborate *v.* 合作；协作	8 Part II A
colon *n.* 结肠	3 Part II A
compass *n.* 范围；范畴；界限	8 Part II A

compassion *n.* 同情;怜悯   6 Part II B

compassionate *adj.* 富有同情心的;怜悯的   7 Part II B

compel *v.* 强迫;迫使;使必须   1 Part II A

compel *v.* 强迫;驱使   7 Part II B

complement *v.* 补充;补足;使完美;使更具吸引力   7 Part II A

compliance *n.* 服从;顺从;遵从   6 Part II A

composition *n.* 组成;成分   3 Part II B

concentration *n.* 浓度   2 Part II A

condition *n.* (因不可能治愈而长期患有的)疾病   8 Part II A

conducive *adj.* 使容易(或有可能)发生的   5 Part II A

conform *v.* 顺从;顺应(大多数人或社会);随潮流   6 Part II A

congested *adj.* 堵塞的   7 Part III

conjunctivitis *n.* 结膜炎   5 Part III

conscientious *adj.* 勤勉认真的;一丝不苟的   5 Part II B

consecutive *adj.* 连续不断的   5 Part I

constrict *v.* (使)紧缩;缩窄   5 Part II B

consultation *n.* (向专家请教的)咨询会;(尤指)就诊   6 Part II A

consumption *n.* 消耗   2 Part II B

contact tracer 接触者追踪人员   1 Part I

contagious *adj.* 接触传染的   1 Part II A

contextual *n.* 上下文的;与语境相关的   7 Part II B

contextualize *v.* 将……置于背景中考虑   7 Part I

continent *n.* 大陆   4 Part II B

contract *v.* 感染(疾病);得(病)   1 Part I

controversial *adj.* 引起争论的;有争议的   5 Part II A

cornerstone *n.* 基石;奠基石   4 Part II A

corporality *n.* 肉体   7 Part II A

cortisol *n.* 皮质醇   5 Part I

cost-conscious *adj.* 注重节约成本的   8 Part II B

courtesy *n.* 礼貌;谦恭;彬彬有礼   8 Part II B

critical *adj.* 关键的   7 Part I

dietary *adj.* 饮食的　　　　　　　　　　　　　　　2 Part III

dilate *v.* 扩大;(使)膨胀;扩张　　　　　　　　　4 Part II A

diminutive *adj.* 微小的;极小的;特小的　　　　　7 Part II A

dimly *adv.* 模糊地　　　　　　　　　　　　　　5 Part III

diphtheria *n.* 白喉　　　　　　　　　　　　　　1 Part II B

discard *v.* 丢弃;抛弃　　　　　　　　　　　　　4 Part II B

disorder *n.* 失调;紊乱;不适;疾病　　　　　　　5 Part I

disparate *adj.* 完全不同的　　　　　　　　　　8 Part II B

disparity *n.* (尤指因不公正对待引起的)不同;不等;差异;悬殊

　　　　　　　　　　　　　　　　　　　　　3 Part II A

disproportionately *adv.* 不成比例地　　　　　3 Part II A

distressing *adj.* 使人痛苦的;令人苦恼的　　　5 Part II A

distribution *n.* 分发;分送　　　　　　　　　　1 Part II B

divide *n.* 差异;分歧　　　　　　　　　　　　　7 Part I

domain *n.* (知识、活动的)领域;范围;范畴　　　7 Part II A

dopamine *n.* 多巴胺　　　　　　　　　　　　　5 Part I

dose *n.* (药的)一剂;一服　　　　　　　　　　1 Part II B

dose-response *n.* 剂量反应　　　　　　　　　2 Part II A

dreaded *adj.* 令人畏惧的;可怕的　　　　　　　3 Part I

dull ache　隐痛　　　　　　　　　　　　　　　4 Part III

dysfunction *n.* 功能紊乱;机能障碍　　　　　　4 Part II A

Ebola *n.* 埃博拉(病毒)　　　　　　　　　　　　1 Part I

ecotherapy *n.* 生态疗法　　　　　　　　　　　5 Part II B

efficacy *n.* (尤指药物或治疗方法的)功效;效验;效力　5 Part II A

elated *adj.* 兴高采烈的;欢欣鼓舞的;喜气洋洋的　5 Part II B

electric current *n.* 电流　　　　　　　　　　　5 Part II A

electrical grid　电力网　　　　　　　　　　　　4 Part II A

electroconvulsive *adj.* 电惊厥的;电休克的　　　5 Part II A

elevate *v.* 提高;使升高　　　　　　　　　　　1 Part II A

elicit *v.* 引起(反应)　　　　　　　　　　　　　4 Part II A

elixir *n.* 灵丹妙药　　　　　　　　　　　　　　2 Part II A

elusive *adj.* 难以解释的；难以捉摸的   2 Part II A

embark on *v.* 从事；着手   5 Part II A

emergency *n.* 紧急情况；突发事件   7 Part II B

empathetic *adj.* 移情的；有同感的；能产生共鸣的   6 Part II A

empathy *n.* 同感；共鸣；同情   6 Part II A

endocrinologist *n.* 内分泌学家   4 Part II A

endorphin *n.* 内啡肽(内分泌激素,有镇痛作用)   4 Part II A

enkephalin *n.* (生化)脑啡肽   4 Part II A

enroll *v.* 注册；加入   7 Part II B

entail *v.* 牵涉；需要；使必要   5 Part II A

entecavir *n.* 恩替卡韦(一种抗病毒药物)   3 Part II B

epidemiologist *n.* 流行病学家   1 Part II B

epigenetic *adj.* 表观遗传学的；后生的   2 Part II B

eradication *n.* 根除；消灭；杜绝   1 Part II B

escalate *v.* 加剧；恶化   4 Part III

evidence-based *adj.* 基于证据的；循证的   5 Part II A

exacerbate *v.* 使恶化；使加剧；使加重   1 Part II A

excessive *adj.* 过度的   2 Part II B

exclusive *adj.* (个人或集体)专用的；专有的；独占的   8 Part II A

expedite *v.* 加快；加速   8 Part II B

expenditure *n.* (精力的)消耗   2 Part II A

exposure *n.* 接触；暴露   1 Part II A

extract *v.* 选取；摘录；选录   8 Part II B

eye drop 滴眼剂   5 Part III

facade *n.* (虚假的)表面；外表   6 Part II B

fasting *n.* 禁食期；斋戒期   6 Part II A

fatigued *adj.* 身心交瘁；精疲力竭   4 Part III

favorable *adj.* 有利的   2 Part II A

feasibility *n.* 可能性；可行性   6 Part II A

fertility *n.* 生育能力；肥沃度   4 Part II A

fertilization *n.* 受精；施肥   4 Part II A

fetus *n.* 胎儿   2 Part II B

filling *n.* 填充;填料   6 Part III

flare *n.* (疾病、伤势)突然复发;突然恶化 1 Part II A

foreign body sensation 异物感 5 Part III

forgo *v.* 放弃;弃绝(想做的事或想得之物) 1 Part II A

formula *n.* 配方;处方;药方 4 Part II B

formulary *n.* (尤指宗教程序或教条的)公式集;配方书 3 Part II A

fracture *n.* 骨折 8 Part III

framing *n.* 构架;框架;构架系统 1 Part II A

free up 释放 4 Part II A

freeze *up* 僵住;陷入困境 5 Part II B

frontal lobe 额叶 5 Part I

gastroesophageal *adj.* 胃食管的 2 Part II B

gastrointestinal *adj.* 胃肠的 2 Part II B

get clear on 弄清楚 6 Part I

gingivitis *n.* 牙龈炎 6 Part III

glaucoma *n.* [眼科]青光眼 3 Part I

glean *v.* 费力地收集;四处搜集(信息、知识等) 6 Part II B

granule *n.* 颗粒 2 Part II B

grapple with *v.* 努力克服 5 Part II A

Guinea *n.* 几内亚 1 Part I

gums *n.* 牙龈 6 Part III

hallucinate *v.* 产生幻觉 2 Part I

hamper *v.* 阻碍;妨碍 7 Part I

hard-to-diagnose *adj.* 难以诊断的 4 Part II B

harrowing *adj.* 令人痛苦的;令人恐惧的 7 Part II B

hassle *n.* 困难;麻烦 3 Part II A

have loose bowels 拉肚子 2 Part III

healthcare facility 医疗机构 1 Part II A

heart and kidney meridians 心经和肾经 4 Part III

heart murmur 心脏杂音 8 Part II B

heart-wrenching *adj.* 令人心碎的;令人痛苦的   7 Part II B

heighten *v.* （使）加强;提高;增加   6 Part II A

heightened *adj.* 加强的;加剧的   1 Part II A

hematopoietic *adj.* 造血的;生血的   1 Part II A

hepatitis *n.* 肝炎   3 Part II B

highlight *v.* 突出;强调   5 Part II A

hippocampal volume 海马体积   5 Part I

hoarse *adj.* 嘶哑的   1 Part III

holistic *adj.* 整体的;全息的   4 Part II B

homoeostasis *n.* 体内平衡   2 Part II A

hormone *n.* 荷尔蒙   2 Part I

hospitalization *n.* 住院治疗   2 Part II B

hum *n.* 嗡嗡声;嘈杂声   5 Part II B

humanoid *adj.* 有人的特点的   8 Part I

humidifier *n.* 湿度调节器   7 Part III

hydration status 水合状态   2 Part II A

hygiene *n.* 卫生   5 Part II B

hyperactivity *n.* 活动过度;极度活跃   5 Part II B

hypertension *n.* 高血压   4 Part I

ibuprofen *n.* 布洛芬   7 Part III

illuminate *v.* 阐明;启发   7 Part II B

imbue *v.* 使充满;灌输;激发（强烈感情、想法或价值）   7 Part II A

imbursement *n.* 支付;报销   3 Part II B

immunity *n.* 免疫力   1 Part II A

immunization *n.* 免疫   1 Part II B

immunocompromising *adj.* 免疫功能受损的   1 Part II A

immunometabolism *n.* 免疫代谢   2 Part II A

impair *v.* 损害;削弱   1 Part II A

impede *v.* 阻碍;阻止   3 Part II A

imperative *n.* 重要紧急的事;必要的事   1 Part II A

impersonal *adj.* 缺乏人情味的;冷淡的   7 Part II A

implement *v.* 使生效;贯彻;执行;实施	6 Part II B
implication *n.* 可能的影响	2 Part II B
imposition *n.* 不公平(或不合理)的要求	1 Part II A
impoverish *v.* 使贫穷;使贫瘠;使枯竭使贫穷	3 Part II B
in line with 符合;与……一致	8 Part II A
in vain 徒劳无益地;无用地	8 Part II A
incentive *n.* 激励;刺激;鼓励	1 Part II B
incidental *adj.* 附带发生的;次要的;非有意的	8 Part II B
induce *v.* 引起;导致	2 Part II A
infamous *adj.* 臭名远扬的;声名狼藉的	6 Part II A
infancy *n.* 婴儿期	2 Part II B
infarction *n.* 梗塞;梗死	3 Part II A
infection *n.* 传染;感染	1 Part II A
inflamed *adj.* 发炎的;红肿的	1 Part III
inflammation *n.* 发炎	2 Part I
inflation *n.* 通货膨胀	3 Part I
influential *adj.* 有影响力的	4 Part II B
influenza *n.* 流行性感冒	1 Part II A
ingredient *n.* 成分	2 Part II B
inhibitor *n.* 抑制剂;阻聚剂	5 Part II A
initiative *n.* 倡议;新方案	1 Part II B
insistence *n.* 坚决要求;坚持;固执	7 Part II A
insomnia *n.* 失眠(症)	4 Part I
intake *n.* 摄入量	2 Part II A
intangible *adj.* 难以形容(或理解)的;不易度量的	5 Part I
integral *adj.* 构成整体所必需的	4 Part II B
interconnectedness *n.* 相互联系;相互关联	1 Part II B
interdisciplinary *adj.* 跨学科的	7 Part II B
interim *adj.* 暂时的;过渡的	3 Part II B
intern *n.* 实习生;住院医生	4 Part II A
interplay *n.* 相互影响(或作用)	5 Part II A

mannerism *n.* 习性;言谈举止   6 Part II A

mantra *n.* 颂歌   2 Part II B

manual *adj.* 用手的;手工的;体力的   8 Part II B

marginalized *v.* 使处于边缘   7 Part I

maternal *adj.* 母亲的   2 Part II B

maternity *n.* 母亲身份;怀孕;产科;孕妇的   3 Part II B

maternity ward 产科病房;产房   8 Part I

matter-of-fact *adj.* 不动感情的;据实的   6 Part II B

mechanism *n.* （生物体内的）机制;构造   2 Part II A

medical bill 医药费   3 Part III

medical circle *n.* 医学界   5 Part II A

medical community 医学界   8 Part II A

medical practice *n.* 医疗实践;医务工作   5 Part II A

medical professional 医疗专业人员   8 Part II A

medicated *adj.* 用药治疗的   2 Part III

medication *n.* 药;药物   7 Part II A

medicinal *adj.* 有疗效的;药用的;药的   8 Part II B

meditative *adj.* 冥想的   4 Part II B

melatonin *n.* 褪黑素   2 Part I

mellow *adj.* 稳健的   8 Part I

menopause *n.* 更年期   4 Part II B

menstrual cramps 月经痛   4 Part I

menstrual *adj.* 月经的   4 Part II A

meridian *n.* 子午线;经线;经脉;经络   4 Part II A

meta-analysis *n.* 元分析   2 Part II A

metaphysical *adj.* 玄学的;形而上学的   4 Part I

metapneumovirus *n.* 偏肺病毒   1 Part II A

metrics *n.* 指标;量度   1 Part II A

micronutrient *n.* 微量营养素   1 Part II B

migraine *n.* 偏头痛   4 Part I

milder *adj.* 更轻微的   5 Part III

milk curd 凝乳 2 Part III

misfire *v.* 不奏效;不起作用 4 Part II A

mitigate *v.* 减轻;缓和 1 Part II A

mitochondrial bioenergetics 线粒体生物能量 2 Part II A

modulate *v.* 调整;调节;控制 4 Part II A

molecular *adj.* 分子的;由分子组成的 8 Part II B

monkeypox *n.* 猴痘 1 Part II B

monotonous *adj.* 单调乏味的 8 Part II A

monumental *adj.* 重要的;意义深远的;不朽的 8 Part II B

morbidity *n.* 发病率 1 Part II A

more often than not 往往;多半 8 Part II A

morning sickness 孕吐 4 Part I

morph *v.* 逐渐变形;转变 7 Part II B

mortality *n.* 死亡数量;死亡率 1 Part II A

moxibustion *n.* 艾灸 4 Part II B

mucous *adj.* 黏液的 2 Part III

multilevel *adj.* 多层次的 3 Part II B

mumbling *n.* 喃喃自语;嘟哝 6 Part II A

mushroom *v.* 迅速增长 1 Part I

mutate *v.* (使)变异;突变 1 Part II B

myocardial *adj.* 心肌的 3 Part II A

myriad *n.* 无数;大量 6 Part II A

nasal congestion 鼻塞 4 Part II B

nausea *n.* 恶心;作呕;反胃 5 Part II A

navigate *v.* 找到正确方法(对付困难复杂的情况) 6 Part II A

nerve *n.* 神经 5 Part II B

neurochemical *n.* 神经化学物质 4 Part II A

neurochemistry *n.* 神经化学 5 Part II A

neurocognitive *adj.* 神经认知的 2 Part II A

neuroimageing *n.* 神经影像 5 Part II A

neurologic *adj.* 神经病学的 1 Part II A

neurologist *n.* 神经科医生　　　　　　　　　　　　7 Part III

neurotransmitter *n.* 神经递质(在神经细胞间或向肌肉传递信息)

　　　　　　　　　　　　　　　　　　　　　　5 Part II A

next of kin　近亲　　　　　　　　　　　　　　　3 Part III

nip sth. in the bud　将……扼杀在萌芽状态;防患于未然　5 Part II B

nitric oxide *n.*　一氧化氮　　　　　　　　　　　4 Part II A

nodule *n.* 节结;小瘤　　　　　　　　　　　　　8 Part II B

non-pharmacologic *adj.* 非药物的　　　　　　　　5 Part II A

norepinephrine *n.* 降肾上腺素;去甲肾上腺素　　　　5 Part I

nosocomial *adj.* 医院的　　　　　　　　　　　　1 Part II A

nourish *v.* 滋养;养育　　　　　　　　　　　　　7 Part II B

nuance *n.* 细微差别　　　　　　　　　　　　　　7 Part I

nutritional *adj.* 营养成分的　　　　　　　　　　2 Part II B

obesity *n.* 肥胖　　　　　　　　　　　　　　　2 Part II B

obsolete *adj.* 过时的;陈旧的　　　　　　　　　　3 Part II B

obstructive *adj.* 梗阻的;阻塞的;栓塞的　　　　　1 Part II A

offspring *n.* 后代　　　　　　　　　　　　　　2 Part II B

olfaction *n.* 嗅觉;嗅诊　　　　　　　　　　　　4 Part II B

oncologist *n.* 肿瘤专家　　　　　　　　　　　　6 Part II A

oncology *n.* 肿瘤学　　　　　　　　　　　　　6 Part II B

onset *n.* 开端;肇始(尤指不快的事件)　　　　　　2 Part II A

optimal *adj.* 最佳的;最优化的　　　　　　　　　4 Part II A

optimize *v.* 使最优化;充分利用　　　　　　　　　6 Part II A

ORS(oral rehydration salt)　补液盐　　　　　　2 Part III

orthodoxy *n.* 普遍接受的观点　　　　　　　　　7 Part II A

orthopedist *n.* 骨科医生　　　　　　　　　　　8 Part III

osteoarthritis *n.* 骨关节炎　　　　　　　　　　4 Part I

outpatient *n.* 门诊病人　　　　　　　　　　　　1 Part II A

overabundance *n.* 过量;过剩　　　　　　　　　4 Part II B

overall *adv.* 一般来说;大致上;总体上　　　　　　5 Part II A

overhaul *v.* 全面改革(制度、方法等)　　　　　　1 Part I

overpacked *adj.* 超载的；负荷过重的   8 Part II A

overprescribe *v.* 处方过量；开(药)过量   5 Part II A

oversee *v.* 监督；监视   1 Part II B

over-the-counter *adj.* 非处方的   7 Part III

pain reliever 止疼药   7 Part III

painkiller *n.* 止痛药   4 Part II B

pale *v.* 显得逊色   1 Part I

pale complexion 苍白的脸色   4 Part III

palpate *v.* 触诊；触摸检查   7 Part II A

palpation *n.* 触诊   4 Part II B

pandemic *n.* (全国或全球性)流行病；大流行病   1 Part II A

parainfluenza *n.* 副流感   1 Part II A

paralysis *n.* 麻痹；瘫痪   1 Part II B

partisan *adj.* (对某个人、团体或思想)过分支持的；偏护的；盲目拥护的

     3 Part II A

parturition *n.* 分娩   2 Part III

pastry *n.* 糕点   5 Part II B

patent *n.* 专利权；专利证书   1 Part II B

pathogenic *adj.* 致病的；病原的；发病的   4 Part II A

pathology *n.* 病理学   6 Part II B

pathway *n.* 途径   2 Part II A

pedestal *n.* (柱子或雕塑等的)底座；基座   7 Part II A

pediatric *adj.* 儿科的；小儿科的   4 Part II A

penalize *v.* 处罚；惩罚；处以刑罚   3 Part II B

penicillin *n.* 盘尼西林(青霉素)   3 Part I

perception *n.* 洞察力；悟性   6 Part II A

pertussis *n.* 百日咳   1 Part II B

pervasiveness *n.* 到处都是的状态   3 Part II A

pharmaceutical *adj.* 制药的   2 Part II B

pharmaceutical *n.* 药物   4 Part II B

pharmacist *n.* 药剂师   1 Part II B

phenotype *n.* 表现型(基因和环境作用的结合而形成的一组生物特征)

2 Part II A

pinpoint *v.* 明确指出;确定(位置或时间)   4 Part III

placebo *n.* (给无实际治疗需要者的)安慰剂   5 Part II A

plight *n.* 困境;苦境   7 Part II B

PMS 经前期综合征   4 Part I

pneumonia *n.* 肺炎   1 Part II A

pockets of 一些   1 Part II B

poignant *adj.* 令人沉痛的;悲惨的;酸楚的   6 Part II B

polio *n.* 脊髓灰质炎   1 Part II B

populace *n.* 平民百姓;民众;人口   3 Part II B

portfolio *n.* (公司或机构提供的)系列产品;系列服务;投资组合

4 Part II A

practitioner *n.* 从业者;执业者   4 Part II B

pregnancy *n.* 怀孕;妊娠;孕期   1 Part II B

preliminary *adj.* 预备性的;初步的;开始的   6 Part II A

premium *n.* 保险费   3 Part II B

prescribing doctor 开处方的医生   6 Part II A

presenteeism *n.* 超时工作   1 Part II A

presymptomatic *adj.* 症状发生前的   1 Part II A

preventive *adj.* 预防性的;防备的   3 Part II A

prioritize *v.* 按重要性排列;划分优先顺序   1 Part II B

privilege *n.* 特殊利益;优惠待遇   8 Part II A

process *v.* 数据处理   8 Part II A

procurement *n.* (尤指为政府或机构)采购;购买   3 Part II B

profile *n.* 概述;简介   5 Part II A

prognosis *n.* (对病情的)预断;预后   6 Part II A

projection *n.* 投射;放映;投影;放映的影像   7 Part II A

promise *n.* 获得成功的迹象   5 Part II A

prospective *adj.* 有望的;预期的;可能的   2 Part II A

protein *n.* 蛋白质   2 Part II B

reuptake *n.* (神经细胞对化学物质的)再吸收;再摄取   5 Part II A

revert *v.* 恢复;回复(到以前的状态、制度或行为)   1 Part II A

revisit *v.* 重提;再次讨论   6 Part II A

revitalize *v.* 使更强壮;使恢复生机(或健康)   1 Part II B

rib *n.* 肋骨   8 Part III

robot vacuum   扫地机器人   8 Part II B

robust *adj.* 强健的;强壮的(体制或机构);强劲的;富有活力的

     3 Part II A

rotation *n.* 轮换;旋转   7 Part II B

rumbly *adj.* 发隆隆声的   5 Part II B

running nose   流鼻涕   1 Part III

saline spray   盐水喷雾剂   7 Part III

SARS-CoV-2   严重急性呼吸综合征冠状病毒 2 型   1 Part II A

savings *n.* 节省物;节省;节约   8 Part II B

savvy *adj.* 有见识的   6 Part II A

scenario *n* 方案;预测   6 Part II A

scour *v.* (彻底地)搜寻;搜查;翻找   6 Part II B

screen *v.* 筛查;检查   8 Part II B

screening *n.* 筛查   1 Part I

sedative *n.* 镇定药   8 Part III

seek out *v.* 挑选出;找出   4 Part II A

self-medication *n.* 自我治疗   2 Part II B

seminar *n.* 研讨会;讲座   7 Part II B

serotonin *n.* 血清素;五羟色胺(神经递质,亦影响情绪等)   5 Part II A

serum sodium *n.* 血清钠   2 Part II A

serve to   有助于   4 Part II A

setback *n.* 挫折;阻碍   6 Part II B

severity *n.* 严重   2 Part II B

side effect *n.* 副作用   4 Part II A

signaling *n.* 打信号;发信号   5 Part II A

significant *adj.* 有重大意义的;显著的   2 Part II A

suboptimal *adj.* 未达最佳标准的;不最理想的;不最适宜的;不最满意的

8 Part II A

subsidize *v.* 资助;补助;给……发津贴　　　　3 Part II B

subsidy *n.* 补贴;补助金;津贴;资助　　　　3 Part II B

suicidal *adj.* 想自杀的;有自杀倾向的　　　　5 Part II A

supplement *n.* 补充物;增补物　　　　2 Part II B

surveillance *n.* 监督;管制　　　　1 Part II A

susceptible *adj.* 易受影响(或伤害等)　　　　5 Part II B

sustainability *n.* 可持续性;可维持性　　　　3 Part II B

swear *v.* 宣誓证明　　　　4 Part I

syncytial *adj.* 合胞体的　　　　1 Part II A

syndrome *n.* 综合征　　　　4 Part II B

synthesize *v.* 综合　　　　8 Part II B

tamp *v.* 压低　　　　5 Part II B

tangible *adj.* 有形的;实际的;真实的　　　　5 Part II B

target *v.* 面向;把……对准(某群体)　　　　8 Part II B

tarnish *v.* 玷污;败坏;损坏(名声等)　　　　5 Part II B

telemedicine *n.* 远程医疗　　　　6 Part II A

temples *n.* 太阳穴　　　　4 Part III

tetanus *n.* 破伤风　　　　1 Part II B

therapeutic *adj.* 治疗的;医疗的　　　　6 Part II A

thorny *adj.* 棘手的;麻烦的;引起争议的　　　　1 Part II B

threshold *n.* 阈;界;起始点　　　　1 Part II A

throbbing pain 通常伴随着心跳或脉搏的悸动感　　　　4 Part III

throw gas on a fire gas 火上浇油　　　　6 Part I

thymopoiesis *n.* 胸腺生成　　　　2 Part II A

thyroid hormone 甲状腺激素　　　　5 Part I

tingly *adj.* 引起(或感到)轻微刺痛的　　　　5 Part II B

tooth extraction 拔牙　　　　6 Part III

tout *v.* 标榜;吹捧;吹嘘　　　　5 Part II B

transcranial *adj.* 经颅的　　　　5 Part II A

transformative *adj.* 变革性的	7 Part II B
transmission *n.* 传送；传递；传达；传播；传染	1 Part II A
treadmill *n.* 枯燥无味的工作(或生活方式)	8 Part II A
trigger *n.* (尤指引发不良反应或发展的)起因；诱因	1 Part II A
tsunami *n.* 海啸；海震	8 Part II A
tuberculosis *n.* 肺结核	1 Part III
tumult *n.* 骚乱；骚动；混乱；喧哗	5 Part II B
underestimate *v.* 低估；对……估计不足	1 Part II A
underinvestment *n.* 投资不足	3 Part II A
underlying *adj.* 根本的；潜在的；隐含的	1 Part II A
underlying imbalance 潜在的失衡	4 Part III
undermine *v.* 逐渐削弱(信心、权威等)；使逐步减少效力	1 Part II B
undetected *adj.* 未被注意的	6 Part II B
unfaltering *adj.* 坚决的	6 Part II A
unfold *v.* (使)展开；打开	7 Part II A
unrelenting *adj.* 持续的；不缓和的；势头不减的	5 Part II B
unstructured *adj.* 结构凌乱的；无条理的；紊乱的；无序的	8 Part II A
upcoming *adj.* 即将发生(或来临)的	8 Part II B
upend *v.* 翻倒；倒放；使颠倒	1 Part II A
uptick *n.* 小幅增加	1 Part II B
up-to-date *adj.* 包含最新信息的；新式的	8 Part II A
usher *v.* 把……引往；引导；引领	5 Part II B
utilitarian *adj.* 实用的；功利的；实惠的	7 Part II A
vaccination *n.* 接种疫苗	1 Part II A
vaccine *n.* 疫苗	1 Part I
vacuum *n.* 真空	4 Part II B
vagus *n.* 迷走神经	5 Part II B
valid *adj.* 符合逻辑的；合理的；有根据的；确凿的	5 Part II A
variant *n.* 变种；变体；变形	1 Part II B
vegetarian *n.* 素食主义者	2 Part II B
vent *v.* 表达；发泄(感情，尤指愤怒)	6 Part I

vessel　*n.*（人或动物的）血管；脉管；（植物的）导管　　　4 Part II A

vial　*n.*（装香水、药物等的）小瓶　　　1 Part II B

viscosity　*n.* 黏稠度　　　4 Part II A

vomiting　*v.* 呕吐　　　3 Part III

vomiting　*n.* 呕吐　　　5 Part II A

vulnerability　*n.* 脆弱性　　　7 Part I

vulnerable　*adj.*（身体上或感情上）脆弱的；易受……伤害的　1 Part II A

waive　*v.* 放弃（权利、要求等）　　　1 Part II B

walk and chew gum at the same time　双管齐下　　　1 Part II B

wasting　*n.* 消瘦　　　1 Part II B

webinar　*n.* 在线研讨会　　　6 Part II A

wheelchair　*n.* 轮椅　　　3 Part III

white-water rafting　乘竹筏漂流　　　5 Part II B

will　*v.* 立定志向；决心；决意　　　6 Part II B

workout　*n.* 锻炼　　　5 Part II B